MENO_

A One-Stop Resource for Feeling Good

Ramona Slupik, M.D., F.A.C.O.G., with Lorna Gentry
With contributions from Cynthia Worby, MSW, MPH, RYT;
Rosemary Clark; Donald Vaughan;
Maureen Ternus, M.S., R.D.; and Kitty Broihier, M.S., R.D.

Adams Media
Avon, Massachusetts

Published by
Adams Media, an F+W Publications Company
57 Littlefield Street, Avon, MA 02322. U.S.A.
www.adamsmedia.com

ISBN: 1-59337-117-9

Printed in Canada.

J I H G F E D C B A

Library of Congress Cataloging-in-Publication Data
Slupik, Ramona. Menopause / Ramona Slupik with Lorna Gentry.
p.   cm.
"Portions of material adapted and abridged from *The everything menopause book*
by Ramona Slupik with Lorna Gentry"—T.p. verso.
ISBN 1-59337-117-9
1. Menopause—Popular works. I. Slupik, Ramona.
Everything menopause book. II. Gentry, Lorna. III. Title.

RG186.S6697 2004
618.1'75—dc22

2004013552

Contains portions of material adapted and abridged from *The Everything® Menopause Book* by Ramona
Slupik, M.D., F.A.C.O.G., with Lorna Gentry, © 2003, Adams Media. Some additional information
adapted from *The Everything® Yoga Book* by Cynthia Worby, MSW, MPH, RYT, © 2002, Adams Media; *The
Everything® Meditation Book* by Rosemary Clark, © 2003, Adams Media; *The Everything® Anti-Aging Book* by
Donald Vaughan, © 2001, Adams Media; and *The Everything® Vitamins, Minerals, and Nutritional Supple-
ments Book* by Maureen Ternus, M.S., R.D., and Kitty Broihier, M.S., R.D., © 2001, Adams Media.

This publication is designed to provide accurate and authoritative information with regard to the subject
matter covered. It is sold with the understanding that the publisher is not engaged in rendering legal,
accounting, or other professional advice. If legal advice or other expert assistance is required, the services
of a competent professional person should be sought.

—From a *Declaration of Principles* jointly adopted by a Committee
of the American Bar Association and a Committee of Publishers and Associations

This book is intended as a reference volume only, not as a medical manual. The ideas, procedures,
and suggestions in this book are intended to supplement, not replace, the advice of a trained medical
professional. Consult your physician before adopting the suggestions in this book, as well as about any
condition that might require diagnosis or medical attention. The authors and publisher disclaim any
liability arising directly or indirectly from the use of this book.

Interior yoga photos by Ron Rinaldi Digital Photography.
Interior flower photos ©PhotoDisc, Inc.

This book is available at quantity discounts for bulk purchases.
For information, please call 1-800-872-5627.

$\mathscr{C}$ontents

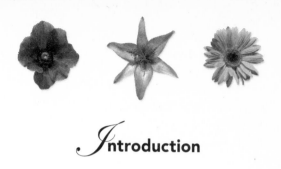

$\mathcal{I}$ntroduction

There are approximately 63 million women over the age of forty in the United States today. As people continue to live longer, healthier, and more active lives, there is much to look forward to: Midlife can be the most productive, enjoyable time in a woman's life.

Hopefully, your career is more established, your children are growing up and becoming more independent, and you're developing a clearer, more confident sense of who you are.

Still, there's no denying that many important and dramatic personal, physical, and psychosocial changes take place as women grow through their forties and fifties. Each woman's journey toward menopause is unique; no two women experience the same feelings or symptoms during this time. And yet, you're certainly not alone if you're reaching this stage in life. Today, most perimenopausal and postmenopausal women are part of the Baby Boom generation—the largest generation in American history. As this sizeable, influential generation reaches middle age and goes through the transition of menopause, it's carrying the rest of our culture with it.

Until the last twenty years or so, very few studies had been done on menopause. Today, however, there is a tremendous amount of information available. Sure, this makes you lucky in one sense, because you have more options and knowledge at your fingertips. But this wealth of information can also seem overwhelming. How do you know which medical studies to believe, which course of treatment to follow, or how to manage your health during menopause when new reports are issued nearly every day?

Think of this book as your filter—your one-stop source for distilling all things menopause-related. In its pages, you'll find simple, straightforward chapters filled with step-by-step advice to help you navigate everything from coping with hot flashes and weighing the pros and cons of HRT, to adapting your nutritional and exercise routine to fit your changing needs and understanding your new sense of sexuality. You'll learn how to help your partner get through menopause, too (that's right, even men can experience their own form of menopause).

Little was discussed about menopause in generations past. The old school of thought treated menopause like a fairy-tale monster that feeds on fear: Menopause exists only in the imagination and, therefore, the best way to overcome it is by denying its existence. But ignoring something doesn't make it go away. These days, doctors—and women themselves—are acknowledging the challenges *and* the opportunities menopause brings more readily. One of the most important things you can do to ensure a healthy transition through menopause is to communicate openly with those around you. Don't be afraid to talk honestly to your health-care provider, share what's going on with your family and friends, and ask for help when you need it. Most importantly, cut yourself some slack. The experience of menopause—just like everything else in life—is a work in progress. Every day will offer new challenges, but also new insights and opportunities, if you're open to them.

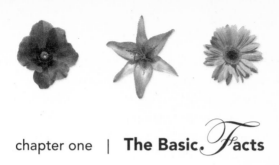

chapter one | **The Basic Facts**

Although menopause is a major life transition filled with both challenges and opportunities, it's not something that hits all at once, making a grand entrance one day out of the blue. For most women, it comes as a series of physical, mental, and emotional changes—some subtle, some more dramatic—which emerge, evolve, intensify, and fade over a period of time. There is no single template for the "typical" menopause profile—every woman's experience is unique. So how do you know when you are approaching menopause? For starters, it helps to understand the basic facts.

What Menopause Is—and Isn't

According to the Council of Affiliated Menopause Societies (CAMS), menopause is "the permanent cessation of menstruation resulting from the loss of ovarian follicular activity." To put it simply, when you have your last period, you go through menopause. Because your periods may become less regular and occur at greater intervals as you approach menopause, however, you don't know you've gone through it for sure until twelve months after your last period.

Natural Versus Induced Menopause

The onset of menopause occurs in different ways:

- Natural menopause, described above, is diagnosed when a woman has had twelve months of amenorrhea (no periods) that is not the result of other physical or pathological conditions or treatments.
- Surgical or induced menopause occurs when a woman no longer menstruates as a result of having her ovaries surgically removed (with or without a total hysterectomy) or when ovaries stop functioning, either temporarily or permanently, as a result of chemotherapy, radiation, drug therapy, or other medical treatments.

Chemotherapy—the use of drugs to treat cancer—may not result in immediate menopause, but it can damage the ovaries. Depending upon the types of drugs used, a patient's ovaries might recover and function normally some time after treatment ends. Sometimes, however, chemotherapy damages ovaries so severely they cannot produce adequate amounts of hormones. In those cases, menopause may occur months or even years after the therapy has ended.

Hysterectomy Doesn't Always Equal Menopause

Having a hysterectomy doesn't mean you'll go through menopause. If your uterus is removed but your ovaries remain, your body will continue to produce hormones. In this case, you don't experience menopause as a result of your surgery, even though you won't have monthly menstrual bleeding.

Pelvic radiation therapy can cause permanent ovarian failure (and, therefore, premature menopause) when the ovaries are near the target of high doses of radiation, for example, as treatment for some types of cervical or endometrial cancer. If ovaries receive only low doses of radiation, they're likely to recover full function.

Because the onset of induced menopause is abrupt, those women have no gradual adjustment period to prepare for postmenopausal changes. Women who have had both ovaries surgically removed, for example, may experience dramatic, abrupt menopausal symptoms, such as severe hot flashes or vaginal dryness.

What Causes Menopause?

The average woman has about 400 reproductive cycles during her lifetime. In every cycle, the woman's pituitary gland produces follicle-stimulating hormone (FSH). This hormone triggers the follicle cells that surround developing eggs in the ovary to produce estrogen. This, in turn, prepares an egg (usually just one) for fertilization. As the body's level of estrogen increases, the pituitary gland stops producing FSH and starts producing luteinizing hormone (LH), which causes the ovary to ovulate (release the egg) and produce progesterone, which prepares the uterine lining to accept the fertilized egg.

The mature egg is only one of several "candidates" available each month. The body then reabsorbs those eggs that don't mature (develop enough to be available for fertilization). If the mature egg is unfertilized, it, too, is reabsorbed and the lining of the uterus is shed in the normal menstrual flow. The body's level of estrogen dips, which then triggers the FSH production that starts the whole cycle again.

As you near menopause, your egg supply diminishes, your follicle cells stop responding to FSH, and you stop ovulating. As a result—over a period of years—you stop menstruating and your ovaries stop making estrogen and progesterone. You may continue to have menstrual periods after you stop ovulating, since your body continues to produce some estrogen. Most women notice a change in the frequency, duration, and flow of their periods during the three to four years before they stop menstruating completely. That's why you can't truly know that you've gone through menopause until a full twelve months after your last period.

What Menopause Means for Your Hormones

Your body produces dozens of hormones, but three of them play a major role in your reproductive cycle: estrogen, progesterone, and small quantities of androgens (testosterone, for example). Here's what those hormones do:

- **Estrogen** is a growth hormone that stimulates the development of adult sex organs during puberty; helps retain calcium in bones; regulates the balance of "good" and "bad" cholesterol in the bloodstream; and aids other body functions, such as blood sugar level, memory functions, and emotional balance.
- **Progesterone** balances the effects of estrogen by aiding the maturation of body tissues and limiting their growth; stimulates the uterus, breasts, and fallopian tubes to secrete nutrients necessary for the body to prepare for growing an embryo and bearing a child; and raises body temperature and blood sugar levels.
- **Androgens** are male hormones produced in small quantities by the ovaries and adrenal glands. The greatest quantities occur at the midpoint of a woman's cycle and may contribute to a healthy libido by fostering a desire for sex.

Many women incorrectly believe that their bodies stop producing estrogen when they stop ovulating. As your ovaries' supply of healthy egg-producing follicles diminishes, the follicles that remain become less potent and produce lower amounts of estrogen. In perimenopause (the time preceding menopause), cycles become less regular and some ovarian follicles don't mature to ovulation; when that happens, the body's level of progesterone drops.

When the pituitary gland senses that the ovaries aren't producing normal levels of hormones, it produces higher levels of FSH, to nudge the ovaries into coughing up more estrogen. In the early stages of perimenopause, that encouragement works; the follicles give up high doses of estrogen, but the body still isn't producing the progesterone that normally rounds out the body's reproductive hormone mix. As a result, a woman in perimenopause may experience widely fluctuating levels of estrogen for a number of years, until the ovaries shut down completely.

When estrogen levels become so low that the lining of the uterus is unable to grow, menstruation stops. The body's FSH levels rise and remain high throughout the postmenopausal years. The body continues to produce small amounts of estrogen, but in levels too small to support the hormone's age-defying functions in the body.

The Stages of Menopause

When we talk about the stages of perimenopause and menopause, we're really talking about the normal aging process—a subject that's become nearly taboo in our youth-oriented Western culture. Fortunately for America's burgeoning post-fifty population, we're living longer, healthier lives today. Thanks to medical advancements, hitting age fifty is now a midway marker rather than a downswing into later life as it used to be.

Remember, menopause is merely one event in the long journey women make as they move away from their reproductive years and into their postreproductive years.

This transformation takes place in stages that occur, for most women, over a period of decades. The following sections detail each of these stages.

The Phases of Menstruation

Women in their teens, twenties, and early thirties who have typical reproductive functions experience monthly menstrual cycles. Some people label these years as "the reproductive years," but it's important to remember that as long as you ovulate and have periods, you are fertile and you can conceive. For the purposes of this book, therefore, just think of this life stage as your early adulthood, which lasts, for the average woman, into her forties.

By the time most women reach their late teens, they ovulate regularly, and their bodies establish their "normal" reproductive cycle. Although the length and regularity of the cycle varies from woman to woman, think of the typical reproductive cycle in terms of two main phases:

- **Buildup (follicular phase)**, the time when one of the ovaries begins developing an egg for release, starting on the first day of menstrual bleeding and continuing until midway through the cycle when ovulation occurs.
- **Premenstrual (secretory phase)**, the time following ovulation when the uterine lining develops in preparation for nourishing a potential fertilized egg.

Hormones trigger each event that occurs during the two phases of one complete menstrual cycle. Here's a rough overview of what happens:

1. On Day 1 of the menstrual cycle, the body begins to shed its built-up uterine lining. The pituitary gland releases follicle-stimulating hormones (FSH) that prompt the ovaries to produce estrogen in order to prepare an egg for ovulation, which develops in one follicle in one ovary. (Occasionally more than one egg matures in the same cycle.)

2. FSH levels pulse occasionally through the next thirteen days as estrogen levels gently rise to their peak.

3. Around Day 14 the pituitary gland releases luteinizing hormone (LH) to make the ovary release the egg and to turn the follicle cells that surrounded the egg into a progesterone-producing machine.

4. For the next two weeks or so, estrogen production slowly diminishes as progesterone production steps up. The two hormones work in conjunction to spur the lining of the uterus to thicken in preparation for accepting and nourishing the fertilized egg.

5. Toward the end of the cycle (around Day 28), the egg reaches the uterus. If fertilized, the egg embeds in the lining and estrogen and progesterone levels remain strong. If the egg is unfertilized, all hormones—FSH, LH, estrogen, and progesterone—drop to minimum levels and the lining of the uterus begins to fall away as menstrual flow, which takes us back to Day 1 of the cycle.

This cycle may take twenty-one days in some women or as many as thirty-five days in others. Studies have shown that your age may play a critical role in the length of your menstrual cycle. Keep a menstrual calendar, and if your cycles fall outside this range, you should discuss it with your doctor.

Fast Facts about Premenstrual Syndrome

Even when you've established your own individual cycle and are in the height of your reproductive years—from your late twenties through mid-thirties—your monthly cycle may not always proceed smoothly. Most women experience some symptoms associated with their menstrual periods, including cramps, swollen and tender breasts, mood shifts, and headaches. Some research indicates that premenstrual syndrome (PMS) can include as many as 150 separate systems, but all symptoms of PMS fall into two major categories:

- **Physical symptoms** include bloating, water retention, pelvic pressure or cramping, and headaches or migraines.
- **Emotional symptoms** can consist of irritability, mood swings, difficulty concentrating, and food cravings.

Some women never have PMS, while others—some studies estimate one-third of all women—may have episodes of it throughout their adult lives. These women often find that PMS is most frequent and severe during their thirties. Many women who have never experienced PMS or have had only occasional, minor symptoms, report severe PMS phases as they enter perimenopause.

Symptom Severity

Don't read too much into new and more severe PMS symptoms. Although they can signal that your reproductive system is slowing down—and that means that you're moving into perimenopause—they can also signal a new awareness of your body or your body's reaction to life's increasing stresses.

A less common but even more debilitating type of premenstrual syndrome is premenstrual dysphoric disorder (PMDD). Women who suffer from PMDD often experience severe depression, anxiety, sleep disturbances, and fatigue in addition to a wide range of physical disturbances. Though these two syndromes differ in severity, diagnosis, and treatment, both seem to be linked to the way the body processes and responds to reproductive hormones.

Doctors diagnose PMS and PMDD based on when a woman's symptoms occur, not just the symptoms themselves. If you want to track your own premenstrual symptoms, you can keep a menstrual journal (see Chapter 3). If symptoms repeat at specific intervals, they may indicate PMS.

The Journey Through Perimenopause

During perimenopause you may experience the classic symptoms, including irregular and/or heavy periods, mood swings, hot flashes, weight gain, and headaches. Or you may experience increased severity of PMS symptoms. PMS and some symptoms of perimenopause mirror each other because both are thought to be caused by fluctuating levels of reproductive hormones. Some women are more sensitive to these fluctuations than others, which explains why certain individuals have no symptoms, while others have severe symptoms.

Talk to Your Doctor

When your perimenopause symptoms cause a great deal of disruption in your life, it's time to talk to your doctor. Doctors can test for conditions of perimenopause by checking hormone levels in your blood. (Newer saliva tests are currently being developed, but most medical experts don't yet consider them reliable.) Those tests may check for levels of estrogen, FSH, and LH—your doctor determines which hormones to check, based on your symptoms and health history. Rising levels of FSH, for example, can indicate that the body is ovulating less frequently, and therefore FSH is being released from the pituitary gland in greater quantities to spur the ovaries' estrogen production. Many health-care providers consider an FSH level of forty or above to be a firm indicator that menopause has occurred. FSH levels can fluctuate in perimenopause, so sometimes a single test doesn't provide enough information on which to base a diagnosis.

Premenopause Versus Perimenopause

The term premenopause is no longer used to refer to the years preceding menopause, because all the years of a woman's life that precede menopause are premenopause. Today, perimenopause is used to describe the years when a woman's reproductive system slows down as it approaches menopause.

If you're in perimenopause, you have a number of options, and your health-care provider can help you explore all of them. (You'll learn more about these treatments in upcoming chapters.) Remember, your symptoms may go through a number of changes or even resolve themselves with no treatment at all. In fact, some estimates say that as many as 55 percent of women in perimenopause use no treatment of any kind. In many cases, your body slowly adjusts to its changing hormone levels, and your symptoms remain mild or even unnoticeable. (Unfortunately, most women whose menopause is artificially induced have more pronounced, severe symptoms and are more apt to require hormone replacement therapy or other treatment options.)

Other Physical Changes During Perimenopause

Most of us can expect to experience other physical changes during—and perhaps as a result of—perimenopause. If perimenopause occurs during a woman's forties, for example, here are some of the changes her body might be undergoing:

- Muscles may lose mass easier and become harder to tone during your forties, so your old workout plan may not be enough to maintain the strength and body weight you enjoyed in your thirties. You may need a new workout program; see Chapter 15.

- Bones can start to lose calcium as estrogen levels recede and the body becomes less efficient at absorbing calcium from food. You may need to adjust your diet to include more vitamin D and calcium, or consider taking supplements. See Chapter 9 for more information.

- Eyes become less efficient as the lenses lose elasticity and their controlling muscles weaken, making focusing close-up more difficult. Estrogen helps keep eyes and muscles elastic, so diminishing levels of estrogen contribute to this degeneration; see Chapter 12.

- Skin and hair can begin to thin in response to lowered levels of estrogen; most people start to get some gray hair in their forties. Estrogen also helps maintain the collagen content (the basic protein bridgework) of your skin, thus keeping it youthful and elastic. Your strong ally in the battle against this aging factor is a healthy diet and lots and lots of water. See Chapters 12 and 13 for more information.

- Metabolism slows down during your forties, so weight gain can creep up on you, even if you maintain your previous diet and workout plan. Typical dieting methods are unlikely to work as well for you at this age; maintaining or losing weight may require additional exercise and calorie cutting. See Chapters 13 and 15.

• Propensities for certain conditions such as diabetes and asthma can accelerate during this time, due to changing hormone levels, lowered resistance to stress and infections, and other factors of aging. Medical checkups and health maintenance are more essential than ever at this point. (See Chapters 7, 8, and 9.)

Don't be put off by this list; yes, the aging process does involve physical changes and even some deterioration of your body's systems. But there's never been a time when medicine and health care, public information, and healthy life practices have been better able to contribute to everyone's pursuit of a healthy, active middle age. You have more control than any generation that's preceded you in how quickly or slowly your body loses ground to the aging process. Learn ways to manage the effects of perimenopause and its role in the aging process.

Beware of How Long Symptoms Last

Although PMS symptoms can occur anywhere from midway through your cycle to a few days after you begin your period, no one symptom should ever last more than two weeks. If you have any symptom longer than fourteen days, report it to your doctor. It may be something other than PMS.

Menopause and the Years Ahead

You know you stop having periods when you reach menopause. But what other changes take place as a result of this transition? And what lies ahead?

Your Hormones Postmenopause

After menopause, estrogen and progesterone levels plummet. The specific role of these hormones is treated in Chapter 6, but some of the major postmenopausal side effects are increased bone loss and the drying and shrinking of the vagina (vaginal atrophy). Fewer vaginal secretions are produced when there is no estrogen, so your vaginal wall becomes less lubricated and flexible and more prone to tears and cracking, especially during intercourse. In fact, all of your skin tissue becomes thinner and less elastic, including the muscles that surround your urethra (the opening to the bladder). That's how diminishing hormone levels can contribute to involuntary urine release through stress incontinence.

Your cardiovascular system misses those hormones, too, with their beneficial impact on HDL cholesterol and their inhibiting effect on LDL cholesterol. And just as your arteries become more susceptible to plaque buildup, they begin to narrow and lose elasticity. As a result, estrogen loss can contribute to heart disease.

Another important side effect of plummeting hormones is a rapid advance of the bone loss that began in your forties. In the first five years that follow menopause, women can lose as much as one-fourth of their bone density. Bone fractures that develop as a result of osteoporosis can have life-threatening consequences. This bone loss slows down for most women within a decade or so of menopause, but without supplements or HRT, it continues throughout a woman's life.

Other Postmenopausal Changes

During your fifties and early sixties—the decades immediately following menopause—your body undergoes some inevitable changes resulting from the natural aging process. Again, your body is unique, and so are your family medical history, your lifestyle, and your individual health program. But in general, here are the types of changes many women experience in the years that follow menopause:

- Hearing loss can set in, because ear-canal tissue becomes thinner and drier, and sensory nerves that transmit sounds from the ears to the brain have lost some of their efficiency. Many people have no hearing loss until they are in their sixties, but almost one-third of women over sixty-five report hearing problems. Keep this loss to a minimum by protecting your ears from loud noises. Also get annual hearing checkups, so you know if you reach the hearing-aid stage.

- Joints lose cartilage and natural lubricating fluid with age, and connective tissue becomes less flexible and resilient, making arthritis and other types of joint pain more common in aging women. Exercise and weight control (obesity puts enormous stress on weight-bearing joints) are critical factors in maintaining healthy joints.

- Lungs become less elastic as we hit our mid-fifties, which can contribute to shallower breathing and, therefore, less oxygen in our bloodstream. Get plenty of aerobic exercise to keep your lungs pumping. And, if you're still smoking, quit now!

- The brain loses mass and shrinks slightly with each passing year. Blood flow can be decreased due to atherosclerosis in the coronary arteries, and as a result, women can face impaired cognitive functions as early as age seventy. Keep your body and mind active. Life's pleasures are also your best weapon in keeping your mind alert and agile. Remember, if you use it, you don't lose it.

- Digestion slows down as we reach our sixties, and food moves at a slower pace through our intestines. As a result, many postmenopausal women report problems with constipation. Eat plenty of whole grains, fresh fruit, and vegetables, and drink plenty of water to combat this change in your digestive function (and, you guessed it, exercise).

A Look at What's in Store

Just because you stop having periods and you move into the postchildbearing phase of your life, that doesn't mean you become old as a result of menopause. According to the North American Menopause Society (NAMS), the average age of natural menopause in the Western world is fifty-one. Most American women born after 1950 can expect to live until their mid-eighties, meaning that the majority of menopausal women in the United States today have one-half to one-third of their lives to live after they've gone through menopause.

What menopause *does* mean is that your body is undergoing changes that require your attention. Menopause means you need to learn new ways to remain healthy, strong, and vital. Menopause also brings opportunities to enjoy new levels of freedom and self-awareness. You may find that you don't miss the experience of menstruation at all. You no longer have to worry about becoming pregnant, so sex can take on new depths of pleasure. Menopause is also a marker of your evolving life; its arrival may encourage you to focus new attention and energy inward, and evaluate who you are, what you're doing, and where you want to go next.

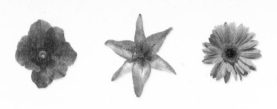

chapter two | **Understanding *Perimenopause***

As stated in Chapter 1, perimenopause is the period of time preceding menopause in which your body's reproductive system slowly winds down. Though perimenopause differs for every woman, it generally marks a time of less-frequent ovulation and fluctuating levels of hormones, including estrogen, progesterone, and FSH. On average, women begin perimenopause at age forty-seven and experience it for about four years. But women can experience some of the symptoms of perimenopause in their late thirties or early fifties, and it can last from a few months to eight or ten years. You have no way of knowing precisely when or how you'll begin noticing the changes that announce you're approaching menopause. Most likely you'll instead connect the dots of a number of odd symptoms and changes that eventually point toward that direction.

Although at first you're likely to have a difficult time accepting that you're perimenopausal, the realization can be a true relief. If you've been having trouble sleeping, experiencing mood swings, feeling anxious, nervous, and depressed, or forgetting things, for example, you might feel like you're losing your mind or developing some odd and difficult-to-diagnose illness. In reality, however, the symptoms you're experiencing are normal, manageable demonstrations of a natural stage in your body's development.

Why Call Them Symptoms?

Don't let the term "symptoms" lead you to believe that this chapter is describing perimenopause as a disease or illness—it's neither. Perimenopause is a natural process of physical change. For the sake of simplicity, this book refers to the body's demonstrations of this natural process as "symptoms," with no connotation of illness or disease.

Consider this chapter your perimenopause orientation session. When you're aware of the range of symptoms women report during perimenopause, you gain a better understanding of this phase of life. You also learn to recognize symptoms that point to other issues in your physical and emotional health. The goal is to help you feel more comfortable and relaxed as you experience menopause, so you're able to pass through each stage more smoothly and you're ready to deal with any problems you may encounter.

Recognizing Perimenopausal Symptoms

What kinds of symptoms are common—or even possible—during perimenopause, and what do they mean? And how do you know if your symptoms are related to perimenopause or some other part of the aging process?

First, it's important to understand that, if you think it may be perimenopause, it probably is. No one is more familiar than you are with your body's feelings and reactions during your monthly cycles. Women have reported a wide variety of symptoms during and after perimenopause. Remember, some women experience no symptoms at all.

Also keep in mind that everyone can expect to experience some physical and mental signs of aging. As women age, many of their physical changes are triggered or exacerbated by hormonal fluctuations. The good news is, any overt symptom that is associated with or triggered by changing hormone levels can be temporary—and may even be diminished through diet, exercise, or other therapeutic options. And above all, never forget that everyone's path to menopause takes its own unique course.

What Women Experience in Perimenopause

If you start noticing obvious changes in the length of your periods, the intervals between them, or the heaviness of your flow, and you're between the ages of thirty-five and sixty, you should start checking for other signs of perimenopause. But changes in your cycle may not be your first indicator that perimenopause is approaching. Many women report symptoms of perimenopause while their periods remain much the same. Though we all have our own perimenopausal profile, most women feel some or all of the following symptoms as their bodies prepare to stop ovulating:

- Hot flashes
- Vaginal dryness and painful intercourse
- Irregular and/or heavy periods
- Involuntary urine release and bladder urgency
- Insomnia
- Mood swings
- Decreased sexual drive
- Weight gain

- Difficulty concentrating
- Heart palpitations
- Migraine headaches

Add to that list everything from aching joints and muscles to the onset of chin whiskers, and you've only just begun to cover the wide variety of symptoms perimenopausal women report.

If the preceding list paints an ugly picture of perimenopause, it's also important to remember that even among women who experience these symptoms, the effects can be mild, transient, or otherwise unannoying. The following sections take a closer look at the causes of these symptoms so that you have a better idea of what to expect.

Hot Flashes and Night Sweats

Along with irregularities in menses, hot flashes are one of the most commonly reported symptoms of perimenopause. Nearly 75 percent of women who report perimenopausal symptoms list hot flashes among them. Hot flashes can come at any time of the day or night, but when they occur during sleep, they're usually referred to as night sweats.

Not so long ago, many doctors considered hot flashes to be figments of the female imagination. Today, we know that hot flashes are real, physiological responses to the body's declining levels of estrogen.

Hot flashes can be mild or severe, but in general, they involve a fast-spreading sensation of warmth in your neck, shoulders, and face that may last a few seconds or as long as thirty minutes or more. This sensation may begin at the top of your scalp, behind your ears, on your chest, or even across your nose. Many women have also reported flashes occurring across the breasts, below the breasts, or all over the body.

When flashes are brief, they may cause only a slight flush on your face, neck, or shoulders. But when they result in dramatic temperature increases, they can produce profuse perspiration on your upper lip, neck, forehead—or even your entire body. During a severe hot flash, the skin on your face, neck, and scalp may become extremely red, and this flush may take longer to fade than the feeling of "heat" itself. Some women have reported a rapid heart rate immediately before and during their hot flashes; a few women have experienced nausea and/or chills following them. Other feelings of physical discomfort, including tension, anxiety, or nervousness, may also come along with hot flashes.

If you suffer from night sweats, you may experience some loss of sleep. Many women sleep right through their nighttime hot flashes and know of them only when they awake in the morning to find their pajamas or pillowcase slightly damp. However, severe night sweats can produce such intense heat and sweating that sleep becomes impossible. Extended sleep loss can lead to feelings of anxiety, tension, and even depression. But only a few women experience this severity.

Irregular and/or Heavy Periods

Even if your periods have always been as regular as clockwork, you can expect some irregularities to occur in the years preceding menopause. As mentioned earlier, as you get older, you ovulate less frequently. Lags and surges in estrogen and progesterone levels can contribute to unusually light or skipped periods or periods that flow for weeks at a time. Some women experience spotting—or even phases of heavy bleeding—for a few days between periods. In other words, you may find that irregularity becomes the norm in your perimenopausal cycles.

An unusual fluctuation in one hormone can set off a series of unusual fluctuations in others, as your body tries to spur on or hold back the hormone in flux. For that reason, you might have a six-week cycle, followed by a four-week cycle, followed by a six-week cycle with unusually light flow, and so on. (A cycle is the length of time from the first day of one menstrual period to the first day of the next.) Keep a calendar if you do not see a clear pattern. Your body is going through a series of starts and stalls as it attempts to adjust to fluctuating levels of hormones in your bloodstream.

Although heavy periods and ongoing irregular bleeding are not uncommon during perimenopause, they shouldn't go unchecked. Nonstop heavy bleeding can leave you tired, weak, and anemic, making you a prime candidate for any cold, flu, or infection that comes your way. More importantly, heavy bleeding may have nothing to do with simple hormonal ebbs and flows. Between 30 and 40 percent of all women develop abnormal tissue in the uterus, such as fibroids or polyps, which begin to cause problematic bleeding during perimenopause. Heavy bleeding could also be a sign of precancerous conditions or even endometrial cancer. Don't take chances if your irregularities are dramatic—see your doctor. (For complications of the uterus and their treatment, see Chapter 7.)

Mood Swings

Among women who cite symptoms in perimenopause, nearly 50 percent say mood swings are among those that bother them the most. The experiences are as individual as the women who have them, but mood swings tend to take the form of intensified emotional reactions. Sometimes, the swing can take you high, and you feel a particularly strong delight in everything around you. Other times, however, mood swings can plunge you into intense sorrow, despair, anger, anxiety, general depression, or fear. A typical anger response during a mood swing can leave your heart pounding, your face flushed, and your head throbbing. Mood swings can trigger bouts of crying and cause deep, dark feelings of hopelessness. Then, as nasty as they can be, mood swings may pass rather quickly, leaving you feeling a bit shaken and confused by the emotional ride.

Acknowledge Depression

Don't confuse mood swings with depression—feelings of despair, hopelessness, lack of energy, and a diluted interest in life around you—with mood swings. When feelings of despair last more than a few weeks, you should consult your doctor. Untreated depression can damage your health and happiness.

Though mood swings seem to be emotional responses, they can be a direct physical response to the changing hormonal levels in your bloodstream. Many perimenopausal women experience mood swings along with other common symptoms of premenstrual syndrome (PMS), even when those women have never before suffered from PMS symptoms. Those symptoms include a wide range of physical and emotional markers, including gastrointestinal distress, headaches, pains in muscles and joints, fatigue, heart pounding, hot flashes, exaggerated sensitivity to sounds and smells, agitation, and insomnia.

Just as mood swings in perimenopause can have both physical and emotional consequences, the causes of those mood swings can be both physical and emotional. First, consider that many of the symptoms of perimenopause can cause emotional distress. Hot flashes can lead to sleeplessness, fatigue, irritability, and anxiety. Those factors can make you feel angry, isolated, and under siege—and contribute to occasional moodiness and transient depression.

Involuntary Urine Release

Nearly 20 percent of all women over the age of forty-five develop some urinary tract problems. Those problems can include UTIs, stress urinary incontinence (caused by a stressor such as sneezing, coughing, or laughing), and urge incontinence (caused by a bladder spasm that forces urine out, even when the bladder is not completely full).

Because your body produces lower levels of estrogen during the years leading to menopause, the tissues lining the urinary tract can grow thin and more prone to bacterial infection and inflammation. That same lack of estrogen-induced nourishment can weaken the muscles that surround your bladder and urethra. As a result, you experience more UTIs and other urinary tract disorders, a weaker bladder, and less control over urine release. (For more on UTIs, see Chapter 7.)

Urge incontinence is the result of a bladder spasm that forces urine out, even when the bladder is not completely full. These involuntary muscle contractions cause the bladder to release urine in varying amounts. Even though the woman may not feel as though her bladder is full and she needs to urinate, the sight, sound, or even thought of water or urination can cause the sudden reflex need to urinate and an accompanying release of urine.

Stress urinary incontinence is another cause of periodic involuntary urine release. It usually has a specific triggering event, such as a sneeze or cough. Some women release small amounts of urine when they bend over, laugh, or exercise.

Stress urinary incontinence is caused by weakened sphincter muscles, which surround the urethra. It can occur in women of any age. Women who have given birth, especially those who've had very large babies or difficult vaginal deliveries, often experience this disorder many years before they approach menopause. But during menopause, weakening sphincter muscles can contribute to the onset of stress urinary incontinence, even in women who have never experienced it. Obesity and chronic lung conditions that produce a lot of coughing, such as emphysema or cigarette smoking, can also cause or aggravate the condition. Certain strengthening exercises called the Kegel exercises, postmenopausal hormone therapy, and even surgery are just some of the treatments used to combat this disorder. Losing weight and quitting smoking help, too.

Changes in Libido

Everyone has a unique attitude toward sex and sexuality, and certainly, we all differ in our sexual habits and desires. While this undeniable (and delightful!) individuality may seem to contradict any generalizations about how sexual desire can change during menopause, many women do experience certain types of changes during this time.

Many studies—including those of the famous Alfred Kinsey—indicate that both men and women can experience gradually declining sexual desire as they age. Remember, however, that not everyone undergoes a noticeable change in libido during menopause—in fact, many women don't. Still, many women in perimenopause have reported noticeable changes in their level of sexual desire. Some say they have more interest in sex and enjoy it more, while others say their desires have diminished. Others say they find sex increasingly unappealing—even painful. If menopause is the trigger for this change, how can it differ so radically from one woman to another?

To understand the answer to that question, remember that human sexuality is a complex and somewhat mysterious force. Changes in sexual desire are rarely explained by simple answers or attributed to single sources—no matter when those changes occur.

Hormones play a critical role in your body's sexual response.

Estrogen increases blood flow to all of your body's tissues, and it helps keep the walls of your vagina well nourished and healthy. Estrogen also helps maintain normal vaginal secretions and contributes to vaginal moistness and flexibility. As your body's hormone levels fluctuate through perimenopause and then diminish after menopause, you might experience some concurrent decline in sexual desire.

But that's not the whole story. Let's not forget those many women who report that their sex lives improve at this stage of life. The reasons for this not unusual phenomenon are relatively easy to understand. As women move into perimenopause and menopause, they may have more access to quality time with a sexual partner. As children become more independent and then leave the family, interruptions and distractions diminish, allowing sex to be unhurried and spontaneous. After menopause, women can stop worrying about birth control and therefore enjoy lovemaking free from unwanted pregnancy. And the growing self-confidence that comes with maturity can be a real turn-on—to both the woman and her partner.

Weight Gain

Weight gain is common as people of both sexes age—that isn't exactly new information. The term "middle-age spread" was coined decades ago to describe the body's tendency to pack on excess weight post-forty. Now, not everyone gains weight during perimenopause or after menopause, and not everyone who does gain weight gains debilitating amounts. But the fact is that the majority of women report weight gain at this time. Even women who don't gain weight may experience a change in their body shape. Many women in middle age gain softer, rounder abdomens, larger hips, thicker waistlines, and even extra weight on their shoulders, arms, and thighs.

Your body's metabolism changes as you move into middle age. As you age, your body burns calories much more slowly (some studies say by as much as 4 to 5 percent) as each decade passes. Instead of burning off the calories that you eat, your body converts them into fat. Your body's furnace just needs less fuel to perform the same functions.

Although you may feel as though you are always on your feet and very active, many people slow down a bit as they move into middle age—running fewer errands, doing less physical work around the house, and so on. All of these factors contribute to unwanted—and sometimes unhealthy—weight gain during perimenopause and after menopause.

Difficulty Concentrating

Though perimenopausal and menopausal women commonly complain of fuzzy thinking, forgetfulness, difficulty concentrating, and memory problems, these issues are linked as closely with the aging process as they are to changing ovarian functions.

This fuzzy thinking often manifests itself in ways you've probably experienced most of your life: for example, losing your car keys, forgetting what you were about to say, recognizing a face but failing to recall the name, searching fruitlessly for the right word, being easily distracted, or losing your train of thought. As women reach the age of menopause (around age fifty), however, they can suffer an increase in these sorts of problems.

Estrogen and Memory

Some studies have shown that estrogen can help heal damaged neurons and increase other neurotransmitters that govern memory and other mental functions, but other studies haven't supported these results. Studies continue, so watch for developments.

The aging process affects the brain, as it does all the other parts of the body.

While you can't stop your brain's odometer from registering the passing years, you can slow down and repair many of the issues that contribute to fuzzy thinking and other cognitive roadblocks. See Chapter 12 for more information.

Heart Palpitations

Heart palpitations are the sudden uncomfortable awareness that your heart is pounding, often at a more rapid rate than normal. Heart palpitations can be frightening, but remember, they aren't uncommon. Certainly, perimenopausal and menopausal women aren't the only ones to experience palpitations—many men and women have them after exercising, when frightened, or while taking some medications. But at menopause, the instances of heart palpitations seem to rise in women. Their frequency and severity vary from woman to woman, but under normal circumstances they aren't a problem. If they get out of hand, however, occurring in rapid succession, heart palpitations can cause problems.

Persistent Palpitations

If your heart palpitations are severe or produce significant discomfort or side effects, you need to talk to your doctor or health-care provider about them. Some palpitations are a warning sign of an impending heart attack. Pay attention to the number and frequency of your palpitations, and be prepared to discuss these and your heart history when you talk with your doctor.

Women describe heart palpitations differently, but in general a heart palpitation feels like your heart is beating rapidly, out of sequence, too strenuously, or in some other abnormal fashion. Some heart palpitations involve only a brief fluttering that passes a few seconds. Other, stronger palpitations can feel like a distinct pounding in your chest that lasts a few minutes and can leave you feeling lightheaded or short of breath.

Anxiety and other system-stimulating problems, such as too much caffeine or an overactive thyroid gland, can also cause palpitations. High or low blood sugar levels can contribute as well. Palpitations that are present upon awakening are particularly worrisome. As you move into perimenopause, your body's fluctuating hormone levels can prompt all of these causes. The good news is that heart palpitations associated with perimenopause and menopause tend to run their course and cease once the body adjusts to postmenopausal hormone levels.

Migraines and Other Headaches

Migraines are intensely painful headaches thought to be associated with constricted blood vessels in the brain. Technically, migraine headaches aren't considered a symptom of menopause. Nevertheless, many women who've never experienced a migraine in their lives begin having them at this point. Younger women often experience these hormonally related migraines in the few days before their periods. In both cases, fluctuations in your body's estrogen levels seem to be a cause.

Though both sexes suffer from migraines, women are three times more likely to have them. Women who suffer migraines describe them as pounding headaches that can cause nausea, vomiting, and a strong sensitivity to light, noise, and odors. Some migraine sufferers—almost one-third, according to some studies—report a certain premonition, or aura, for several minutes before the actual pain begins. This aura can include flashing lights, certain odors, changes in their vision, or numbness in a hand, arm, or leg. Migraines usually last four or more hours, and they can last as long as a week.

Migraines aren't the only kind of headaches that seem to accompany perimenopause. In general, women report having more frequent and severe headaches during this time. These are usually simple stress or muscle tension headaches, and over-the-counter analgesics such as aspirin and acetaminophen often relieve them. If you have a bad headache that lasts more than twenty-four hours, or if it's very severe and lasts for more than a few hours, report it to a doctor. If you have tried to take OTC meds and have no relief, call your doctor or go to the emergency room; you may be in the process of a stroke or ruptured aneurysm.

Insomnia

Perimenopausal and postmenopausal women commonly complain of interruptions in normal sleep patterns. During the years approaching menopause, many women find that they wake once or twice during the night and then have a difficult time returning to sleep. Other times, women find that it takes longer for them to fall asleep when they go to bed at night or that they awaken an hour or two earlier than they used to. Whatever form it takes, insomnia leaves women feeling tired, irritable, and out of touch with their surroundings.

As we age, most people establish new sleep patterns. Although some women go through a phase during perimenopause in which they actually require more sleep than they have previously, others experience periods of wakefulness and restlessness during hours that they previously would have been deeply asleep. Stress, changes in diet, the need for frequent urination, heartburn, hot flashes, and anxiety are a few of the different factors that can trigger insomnia. And, the factors that prevent you from falling asleep when you first go to bed at night can be very different from those that wake you and keep you awake in the middle of the night.

Fortunately, many women find that insomnia is a transient problem that may last no more than a few months. For others, insomnia during perimenopause may be so severe that it hampers their performance and sense of well-being during the day. Chapter 10 offers a number of good options for minimizing insomnia when it strikes. As always, if your symptoms become severe, consult your doctor or health-care professional. You can combat insomnia, so don't allow it to drag you down during this important transition phase.

Preventing Insomnia

Most health-care professionals agree that certain lifestyle habits can contribute to insomnia—at any time in your life. Get regular exercise and try not to consume any alcohol, sugar, caffeine, or rich foods within the two to three hours before bedtime.

Stay on Top of Your Symptoms

Be certain that you are doing all you can to maintain peak health during this important time of transition, pay close attention to your body, and don't ignore the messages it sends you. Many of the symptoms that initially seem par for the course for middle age may be symptoms of problems requiring serious and quick medical treatment. Don't ignore any ongoing problem because you think it's just the change. Work closely with your health-care provider to make sure that your body gets any and all of the help that it needs to stay strong, fit, and healthy.

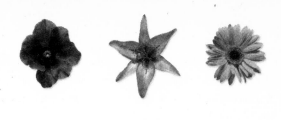

chapter three | *Finding the* **Right Fit with a Doctor**

In an age of HMOs, PPOs, and a never-ending string of traditional and alternative health-care providers, few women go through their adult lives with a single practitioner. The increased mobility of modern life has served to do away with the lifetime family doctor, too. Every woman needs to become an active member of her health-care "plan" by working closely with her primary care provider. This becomes especially important when you're approaching menopause, because you require some special qualities in a health-care provider. If you have been a passive patient up to this point, now's the time to get serious and get involved in ensuring your good health throughout menopause—and beyond.

Your Changing Medical Needs

During perimenopause and menopause, your health-care needs differ from when you were younger. You may begin experiencing abnormalities in your menstrual cycle. Your symptoms could be caused by hormonal fluctuations—or by serious diseases, such as precancerous changes in the lining of the uterus or even endometrial cancer. You may need diagnosis and treatment of emotional as well as physical symptoms. And you most certainly will need the medical advice of someone who is up-to-date on medical advancements in menopause symptoms and treatment.

You may have a great health-care provider right now, or you may need to begin your search for the doctor that's right for you. In either case, now is the time to evaluate what you want and need in a health-care provider and to make sure that you've found the person who fulfills that role.

Finding the Right Qualities in a Health-Care Provider

When you're choosing a health-care provider, medical or professional licensing and board certification are a must, of course. But beyond that, what qualities matter most to you in a health-care professional? Maybe you've been used to gruff, no-nonsense doctors in the past, but now you need a doctor who's willing to listen to your fears, questions, and concerns—one who will encourage you to take an active role in managing your health-care options. Or perhaps in the past you've been content with the variability of a large local clinic or service, but now you're looking for more personalized, in-depth health-care testing and treatment.

Sticking with Your Primary Care Physician

If both you and your primary care physician (PCP) are comfortable with the arrangement, there's no reason for you to see a specialist during menopause. If you have severe or unusual symptoms, however, your PCP is likely to refer you to a specialist for diagnosis and treatment. Talk to your PCP about his or her recommendations for your health care during menopause.

The first step in choosing the right health-care provider for your menopause journey is to determine the kind of person with whom you want to work.

Ask yourself these questions:

- Do you prefer to see a male or a female health-care professional? You need to be comfortable with this person, so decide if gender plays a role in your willingness to discuss symptoms, lifestyle factors, and treatment alternatives.
- Do you feel comfortable with a medical "boss" who dispenses advice and guidance without requesting your input? Or would you prefer someone who is open to the patient-as-partner approach to health care? There's nothing wrong with expecting your health-care provider to suggest specific treatment options— as long as that person is fully trained and has a complete understanding of your medical background and family history. If, on the other hand, you want to choose from a range of options, you need to be certain that your health-care provider is willing to discuss options with you and support your decision with good follow-through treatment.
- Do you care about the age of your health-care worker? Again, it's important that you feel comfortable, you're willing to discuss your health and lifestyle issues openly, and you're confident in the decisions and recommendations offered.

Professional Qualifications

When considering medical care specifically for your treatment during menopause, first decide what kind of special training you want your caregiver to have. If you want someone with specialization beyond that of a general practitioner (GP), you can choose among several types of traditional and nontraditional options. Within the realm of traditional medicine, here are some of your choices:

- An obstetrician/gynecologist (ob/gyn) is specially trained in prenatal care for expectant mothers, the delivery of babies (the obstetrician part), and care of women's reproductive health from menarche to menopause and beyond (the gynecologist services). With the menopausal population booming, more ob/gyns are specializing in menopause. These specialists remain up-to-date on menopause symptoms, testing, treatment methods, and new developments in the use of HRT.

- A reproductive endocrinologist is a doctor who specializes in hormone imbalances and infertility. Since these physicians focus on reproductive hormones, they are likely to remain current on HRT and other treatments and issues that impact menopausal women. Some of these physicians deal strictly with infertility issues, so check before you make the appointment.

- A nurse practitioner is a Registered Nurse (RN) who can perform physical examinations, diagnose and treat illnesses and injuries, prescribe medication, and provide other health-care functions. A women's health nurse practitioner (WHNP) has special training in the area of women's health. Recent studies have shown that many people of both sexes are choosing nurse practitioners as primary health-care providers because of the amount of time they spend discussing health issues and their accessibility to patients.

Alternative health care is big business in the United States. According to an article in *Mayo Clinic Proceedings 2001* entitled "Prevalence and Use of Herbal Products by Adults in the Minneapolis/St. Paul, Minn. Metropolitan Area," 41–62 percent of adults use medicinal herbs. Many women turn to alternative health-care techniques during menopause; here are some of the types of health-care providers they choose:

- Herbal remedies are growing in popularity in Western cultures, and many women today turn to medicinal herbs such as black cohosh, evening primrose, and gingko biloba to offset symptoms such as hot flashes, insomnia, and memory loss. Herbalists are trained to help determine the best types, amounts, and delivery mechanisms for herbal treatment of menopause symptoms, although the data for some supplements may be lacking from a scientific standpoint.
- Homeopaths offer medical treatment based on the principle that "like cures like." Homeopaths prescribe small doses of substances that, if not diluted, would actually make symptoms worse. Homeopathic prescription amounts are based on the severity of symptoms rather than the age and weight of the patient.
- Acupuncturists use a 2,000-year-old Chinese treatment technique that involves rotating fine, sterilized needles into the patient's skin to bring about a therapeutic response. Many women in menopause turn to acupuncture for relief of such symptoms as headache, anxiety, insomnia, and fatigue.

These are just a few of the nontraditional services you can turn to during menopause. Many women use alternative medicine techniques in conjunction with traditional medical health care. If this combined approach appeals to you, make sure you choose a health-care provider who is open to helping you do so.

Once you determine what kind of health-care professional you want, you have a number of options for finding someone in your area whose qualifications match your needs. Beyond asking your family physician or family and friends for recommendations, here are some other ways you can locate a health-care provider:

- Visit the NAMS (North American Menopause Society) Web site at *www.menopause.org* to download a list of health-care providers registered as menopause specialists. The listing indicates licensing and location to help you narrow your search.
- Call reputable medical clinics or teaching hospitals in your area to find out if their Physician Referral services include menopause specialists.
- Check with your insurance provider for a list of doctors and therapists with menopause specialties. Most health insurance companies have Web sites listing physicians in your area or affiliated with major hospitals.
- Search online for menopause specialists in your area using any of the major search engines such as Google, Northern Light, or Excite.

Once you've narrowed the list of potential health-care providers, dig deeper to find out if their operation meshes well with your needs and preferences. Follow a few practical guidelines for screening candidates:

- Call the office, and pay attention to the details. Is the office big and busy or small and personal? Are you immediately put on hold, and if so, how long do you wait? Can the receptionist answer your questions or put you in contact with someone who can? What are the office hours? How does the doctor or practitioner handle emergency calls? How long will it take for you to get an appointment? What's the length of an average office visit? (You want to have adequate time with the doctor or practitioner.) Can patients get responses to questions over the telephone or through e-mail? If so, who returns those calls or e-mails?

- Find out what kinds of insurance the office accepts and how insurance billing is handled. Also check with your insurance provider to be certain that any alternative or specialty treatment you receive is covered before you embark on any potentially expensive testing or treatment plan.

- Schedule an information visit with the doctor or practitioner, then use that visit to assess the condition of the office, the helpfulness of the staff, and your impression of the health-care provider. If the doctor or practitioner doesn't limit his or her practice to menopause (and most don't), find out approximately what percentage of the patient load involves menopause treatment.

- Find out if the practice has an office manager or assistant who can answer your questions and help you get the service you need when the doctor or practitioner is busy or away. Some offices have a registered nurse who performs this function, while others use a medical assistant or even a layperson with extensive medical knowledge and training. The title isn't as important as this individual's willingness and ability to help you resolve issues satisfactorily.

Your prescreening efforts are well worth the time and effort you invest in them. The health-care provider you choose will be an important part of your life for several years to come. Choosing the provider who works best for you can make all of your health-care decisions easier and help ensure that you get the best available care, advice, and guidance.

Talk with Your Doctor

Finding a great doctor or other health-care provider is only half of the sound menopause management equation. You need to be an active, informed, involved partner in your health-care program. Don't be passive when dealing with doctors. If you've followed the advice in this chapter, you've spent a lot of time and energy tracking down the right health-care provider. Do yourself and your health-care provider a favor, and approach your consultation as an exchange of information—not a tell-me-what-to-do-and-I'll-leave event. Prepare for your visit so as to use your time effectively. Make a list of questions covering all the items of special concern to you.

Your Doctor's Influence

Choose your health-care provider carefully, because he or she will have a big impact on the decisions you make about therapies and treatment. In one study by a medical researcher from the Harvard Medical School, 96 percent of women in an HMO who had received an initial prescription for HRT cited their doctor's opinion as critical to their decision to pursue that treatment option.

During your initial office visit, the doctor or practitioner will ask you a number of questions regarding your individual and family health histories. You'll need to report on any history of blood clots, heart disease, breast cancer, and osteoporosis, among other conditions. Your doctor or practitioner will also ask you about your current medications—both over-the-counter and prescription drugs—as well as your use of alcohol, recreational drugs, and tobacco. You're not running for class president here, so don't whitewash the facts by presenting yourself as you think you should be. If you drink or smoke, say so. And don't forget that over-the-counter medications such as pain relievers, vitamins, minerals, and nutritional supplements count, too.

Mention all symptoms you've been experiencing—both emotional and physical. If it helps you to remember, take a written list of symptoms, questions, and concerns with you to your visit. Then write down the answers you receive.

Don't be afraid to ask for clarification if your doctor or practitioner uses terminology you don't understand. It's better to ask for clarification immediately rather than call the office back after you've returned home. Many doctors' offices also have preprinted brochures regarding various aspects of menopause, so feel free to ask.

Finally, discuss all treatment options that interest you, regardless of the medical specialization of the health-care provider you've chosen. Ask about specific treatment options for particular symptoms. If you think you might want certain tests that the doctor hasn't actually offered, speak up. Bring up insurance coverage as well. The more you understand about the specific functions and goals of treatment programs, the better able you'll be to decide which plan is right for you (and the more likely you'll be to follow the plan as recommended).

Take an Active Role

In order for any therapy to be effective, you must be committed to following it—as directed—for as long as is necessary. Remember, you aren't a passive observer in your journey through menopause. Being an active partner in your treatment plan involves carefully monitoring your response to therapeutic drugs and treatments and keeping your health-care provider(s) informed of your progress. If you have a negative reaction to drugs or other treatment options, speak up. You could be experiencing normal adjustment reactions or you could be embarking on a plan that simply doesn't match your body chemistry, lifestyle, or biological and physiological makeup. You won't know what's wrong unless you report the reaction to your doctor or practitioner. If you are using a combination of treatment options, make sure that you coordinate all of them with your primary caregiver.

It's often a good idea to seek a second opinion; reflect on all the options you've been offered, and consult the specialist you feel most comfortable with about combining therapies.

If you're unhappy with the health care you're receiving, say so. Your doctor, practitioner, or therapist can't correct a problem that he or she doesn't know about. If you feel that your doctor or practitioner is unresponsive to your questions and concerns, give him or her an opportunity to discuss your feelings. Although you want to build and maintain a respectful relationship with your caregiver, choose honesty over diplomacy in this discussion. Be specific and open as you state your concerns, and listen carefully to your caregiver's response. If you can't resolve your differences, it's time to start looking for another health-care partner.

Keeping a Menopause Calendar/Journal

If you have begun to notice changes in your monthly cycle or other symptoms, your doctor or health-care professional can perform tests to determine whether you're entering this phase. But you can also begin the diagnostic process yourself by keeping a menstrual calendar/journal to record the physical and emotional changes and symptoms you experience each day as you move toward and through menopause. By chronicling your experiences, you'll better understand where you've been—and, perhaps, where you're going.

See What Other Women Have to Say

Interested in seeing what other women write about their experience with menopause? The Discovery Channel hosts one woman's menopause journal online, at *www.health.discovery.com*. Go to Women's Health and search under "menopause journal."

Track Your Symptoms

You can use a desktop calendar, appointment book, wall calendar, electronic calendar file, a journal, or any medium you choose, as long as your calendar lists days and dates and provides room for you to record your daily notes. To save room, devise abbreviations for symptoms and events.

Part of your journal will be a medical record where you include your menstrual periods and list physical observations, such as mood swings, irritability, migraine headaches, irregular periods, insomnia, weight changes, fatigue, forgetfulness, depression, and so on. Also note the severity, frequency, and recurrence of your symptoms. This way, if any associations or patterns exist, you or your doctor will notice.

You also need a rating system to rank the severity of your symptoms so that if, for instance, you have a mild headache one day and a migraine another, you can track the difference. Similarly, you can note how light or heavy your flow was on any day of your period. You may choose to rank severity with a scale of 1 to 5, with 1 being least severe/lightest and 5 being most severe/heaviest. Use this ranking to note your general mood, too. Add new symptoms as they occur to get a full picture of how your health changes.

Finding Time to Write

Like most worthwhile endeavors, journaling takes practice. Write once a day, at the same time, and in the same place every day. Maybe put your journal next to your morning coffee cup or on your nightstand. Over time, you may choose to be freer in your approach to journaling, but when you're just getting started, setting a regular schedule will help you develop the journaling habit. If time is a problem, "automate" as much as possible: Find ways to create spreadsheets, checklists, or other timesaving formats.

Keep the calendar for at least three months to get a good roadmap of recurring symptoms and your cycle's regularity or irregularity. This information can help you—and your health-care provider—spot symptoms that might be associated with perimenopause.

Many women have found that simply tracking and understanding the cyclical nature of their perimenopausal symptoms makes those symptoms less severe and intrusive. For example, if you know that on the twenty-first day of your cycle every month you're prone to feeling anxious or depressed, but the feeling passes by Day 23, those feelings may seem less debilitating. Keeping a menstrual calendar won't cure your perimenopause symptoms, but the more you know, the better able you'll be to make strong, informed decisions about how you respond to those symptoms.

Medical Information to Note

Though your menopause journal is much more than just this list of physical and emotional symptoms, those records are an important source of information for both you and your doctor, so choose them carefully. Your doctor can tell you which symptoms he or she would most like you to track, but here are some ideas to get started:

- **Keep a diet journal:** List the foods you eat, serving sizes, and calorie counts if you're concerned about pinpointing the sources of weight gain or improving your nutrition. Tracking your diet is also a helpful way to uncover connections between the foods you eat and menopause symptoms.

- **Keep an exercise journal:** If you include the exercise you do each day, the length of time you exercise, number of repetitions, and related information, you'll be able to track your progress and note any associations between your exercise, your symptoms, weight changes, and overall feelings of well-being. Quantifying your time, speed, repetitions, and so on can be visually gratifying and another incentive to improve further.

Don't Stop Journaling

Continue your journal after the doctor prescribes any medical or hormonal therapy or if you add an over-the-counter supplement to your regimen, so that you can gauge any positive result or side effects over time.

- **Track all cyclical symptoms:** Many women experience cyclical symptoms as they move through perimenopause. For example, hot flashes, migraine headaches, or insomnia may occur at specific points in the menstrual cycles. Also be certain to note days in which you have extraordinary feelings of calm, optimism, or energy. Don't just be on high alert for negative days; track positive feelings as well.

- **Note changes in medication or supplements:** One entry in your journal should include all of the vitamins and medications you take on a daily basis. Also record any changes from your daily routine, add and remove medications as your prescriptions change or end, incorporate changes in the types or amounts of vitamin and mineral supplements you're taking, and so on.

Your Journal as a Personal Record

You also can use your journal to record your emotional symptoms and responses to the process of passing through perimenopause and menopause. The very act of writing down your thoughts and feelings is a powerful tool for understanding them. Your journal gives you a much closer look at who you are, who you're becoming, what you most fear, and what your hopes for the future entail.

Use Your Journal for Introspection

Many women have noted that perimenopause and menopause trigger feelings of introspection they haven't experienced before. If you find yourself thinking about your past, write it down! Making a record of these thoughts will help you to see what those past events might be saying to you now. Just remember to keep separate medical and personal journals.

Writing in your journal may also provide a means for you to lessen the effects of stress. By writing about what triggers your stress, your reactions to it, and your thoughts about resolving it, you give yourself a moment to stop the cycle of nervous tension, worry, anger, and fear.

Listen Up, Speak Up, Be Honest

Your job's not through after you've chosen a health-care provider who meets your needs and begun keeping track of your symptoms and feelings. You play an ongoing role in helping your health-care provider to give you the best advice and treatment during perimenopause. To ensure a good rapport with your doctor, always remember to follow these important guidelines:

- Don't assume that you already know what your caregiver is going to say—listen carefully.
- Ask questions, voice concerns, report problems, and discuss options; your caregiver depends on your active involvement in your health-care plan.
- Be honest. You can't have a good health-care experience if you don't communicate honestly with your health-care provider.

Finally, don't judge the quality of your menopause specialist by how often that person agrees with you. You want a health-care provider who'll help you pursue a treatment path that's effective and safe. Find someone you can trust, then discuss your concerns and ideas with an open mind, and—if necessary—seek a second or third opinion.

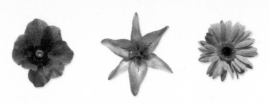

chapter four | **Attitudes and Myths about Menopause**

The way you think about menopause, aging, change, and your own self-worth is all-important at this time of physical and emotional transition. This chapter acknowledges and evaluates some of the "truths" you've learned about menopause and aging over the years and how those ideas can affect your attitude toward your own experience. It also takes a closer look at some of the myths and fears that surround menopause and offers some simple techniques for tracking unproductive and unhealthy beliefs to their source and cleaning them out of your mental closet. It's easy for you to believe the worst about menopause; now, it's time to see menopause for what it is—and what it can be.

We've Come a Long Way

If you ask many women in their fifties today what their mothers told them about menopause, they're likely to respond, "She never mentioned it to me." If society was breaking down the barriers that deemed menopause an unacceptable topic, why wasn't more information available about menopause during the 1970s and 1980s? Much of the lack of new information about menopause during this time was the result of a shortage of good menopause research prior to the last quarter of the twentieth century. And, the research that was being conducted wasn't available to the general public, so many women in the 1970s didn't have access to updated, comprehensive medical information about symptoms, their causes, and how they might be alleviated.

Since the late 1970s, the medical profession has studied menopausal women more than in any time in history, and that has changed the way science and society view menopause. Symptoms such as hot flashes, insomnia, and irritability were once viewed as psychosomatic, all-in-the-head responses to the panic of aging. Today, many scientists trace these symptoms to specific changes in the body's hormone levels. In the 1980s, most women viewed hormone replacement therapy (HRT) as the only option for relieving menopausal symptoms. Today, HRT is just one treatment choice. The world is a different place for today's menopausal women thanks, in part, to data gathered for and by their mothers' generation. The computer age is also responsible for making it easier for almost anyone to access different types of information from a multitude of sources.

Nowadays, menopausal women don't have to "shut up and get through it" or deny that they're experiencing natural emotional and physical reactions to this important passage.

Your Attitude and Why It Matters

At some point, every woman begins to contemplate certain facts about this time of transition and to acknowledge basic truths about the aging process as well as the physical and emotional changes menopause brings. So how do you feel about menopause? Do you dread it? Are you looking forward to the freedom of moving beyond menstruation and into a life free of the possibility of unwanted pregnancy?

Or do you equate fertility with femininity and worry that menopause will leave you dried up and dreary? Are you hopeful that with the right diet, treatment plan, and nutritional supplements you can get back the body you had at twenty-five—or at least keep the one you have at forty-five? Do you know the woman you are, and can you accept the woman you are becoming?

Your attitude toward menopause and the aging process will determine the answers to many of these questions. And the first step in understanding how you feel about menopause is to examine the source of those feelings and ideas.

Menopause Myths

The common wisdom of menopause—the information and misinformation that fuels society's beliefs—plays an important role in determining what we believe. Take a moment to review some of the beliefs that make up the common wisdom of menopause so you can understand the truths—and untruths—they hold.

Myth #1: Menopausal Women Lose Interest in Sex.

The lack-of-libido mythology about women in menopause is part of the common wisdom shared by both men and women—and it's simply not true. A number of studies have shown that only a small percentage of postmenopausal women report a lack of interest in sex, and over half of all women studied report no decrease in sexual interest at all after menopause. (See Chapter 11 on Menopause and Sexuality.)

Myth #2: Women in Menopause Gain Weight, Have Hot Flashes, and Lose Control of Their Emotions.

Lots of people think that the typical woman in menopause is fat, flushed, and out of control. While hot flashes, weight gain, and mood swings are all symptoms reported by some women in menopause, they aren't inevitable side effects. Many women—as many as 10 to 20 percent of women studied—exhibit no symptoms of menopause at all. And while studies show that as many as half of all women in perimenopause experience some weight gain, other women actually lose weight during perimenopause; and many of those who gain weight before menopause lose it afterward. (You'll learn more about these symptoms in other chapters.)

A *Passing* Phase

Although as many as 85 percent of menopausal women report hot flashes, most women find them to be intermittent and, on average, they diminish completely within five years after menopause.

Myth #3: Hormone Replacement Therapy Is Dangerous.

Almost 35 percent of women in menopause use some form of hormone replacement therapy (HRT). It's true that HRT can have dangerous consequences for women with a history of breast cancer, blood clots, endometrial cancer, and certain other family health concerns. No reputable doctor would prescribe HRT for a woman whose health history indicates it may be harmful for her. But most doctors agree that HRT is one of the most effective methods available today for minimizing both the uncomfortable symptoms and health-threatening side effects of menopause.

Myth #4: HRT Is the Only Viable Option for Dealing with the Symptoms of Menopause.

Depending upon the symptoms you experience, simple lifestyle changes may address your most annoying reminders of menopause. During your mother's experience with menopause, HRT was just about the only treatment option discussed with women in the transition. So many women in that generation faced an HRT-or-nothing choice. But the options have changed dramatically over the past thirty years.

Stay Up to Date

To keep up with some of the latest news about HRT, you can search under "Menopause" on the National Library of Medicine's Web site at *www.nlm.nih.gov/medlineplus/menopause.html.*

Myth #5: Menopausal Women Are Angry, Bitter, and Old.

There's a big difference between growing older and being "old." And who has time to be hung up on a numerical age, anyway? It's how old you *feel* that counts. Beyond that, few women in this society have lives that grind to a halt when their reproductive system slows down. Menopause can be a time of unprecedented self-confidence, freedom, and financial liberation for women. Anger and bitterness aren't a natural and inevitable side effect of the transition. However, menopause can also be a time of reflection, introspection, and personal assessment.

If you keep an open mind and pay attention to your own body and the facts about menopause it teaches you, you'll find your own set of common wisdom truths about this transition and what it means for you.

A Brand-New Start

Part of the freedom of menopause is that it gives women an opportunity to define themselves in terms of who they are rather than how well they fit the stereotype of what women can be. Many women spend their youth attempting to fulfill the popular culture's ideal of what a woman should be: thin, beautiful, neat, industrious, helpful, tireless, and supportive of family, friends, supervisor, parents, and anyone else that she encounters in her day. In other words, she's a mother, a wife, and a helper. Women in menopause have an opportunity to throw down that identity and discover what they want, what they enjoy, how they can best fulfill their needs—and learn how to be their OWN best friend and companion as well.

Alternative Options

Alternative treatments are any treatment other than the traditional treatment of hormone replacement therapy. Alternative treatments include anything from vitamins and herbs, to nutritional supplements of soy and phytoestrogens, to cognitive therapy, acupuncture, and biofeedback.

There's no doubt that at times it can be difficult for menopausal women to deal with the changes this phase of life brings. When you're no longer a young mother, a young wife, or the young, new person at the office, you realize that one identity is passing even as another begins. But menopause is not primarily a time of loss; rather, it's a time for every woman to reassess her life, expand in new directions, recognize her changing sense of self, and realize that this evolution is for the better.

Since you were born, you have been in a constant state of growth and change. Through the years, your attitudes and beliefs have helped determine how well you fared in each stage of your life. Your ability to adapt to change, to take advantage of opportunities that came your way, and to capitalize on the realities of your situation have determined the successes or failures you've enjoyed. That's why your attitudes and beliefs about menopause matter. As part of the largest generation of post-fifty-year-old women in our nation's history, you have the opportunity to help shape the common wisdom about what postmenopausal women are all about. Deciding to be well informed and active in the maintenance of your future health and happiness is the surest way toward a good experience with menopause and a healthy, fulfilling postmenopausal life.

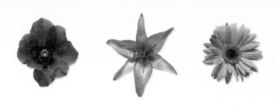

chapter five | **Coping with Hot Flashes**

When women seek relief of menopause symptoms, hot flashes are the symptom they cite most often. Though hot flashes fade over time, severe vasomotor symptoms can disrupt both the waking and sleeping hours of your busy life for several years. Fortunately, you have many options to choose from for reducing or eliminating hot flashes, but you need to choose carefully—and in consultation with your health-care professional.

Nearly 90 percent of all women passing through the stages of menopause will experience hot flashes during some part of the transition. As you learned in Chapter 2, a variety of physical symptoms and sensations can be related to hot flashes. Mild hot flashes pass with little or no impact on general feelings of well-being, while severe hot flashes can last up to forty-five minutes and cause the skin temperature to rise dramatically.

If hot flashes are severe or long-lasting, they can contribute to a number of issues that can have a negative effect on your health and well-being. When hot flashes degrade the quality of your sleep or prevent you from being fully functional during the day, you need to take action.

What's Happening When You Have a Hot Flash?

Hot flashes are connected to changes in your estrogen levels, though the specific cause-and-effect relationship is still under study. Flagging levels of estrogen set the stage for hot flashes, but the actual hot flashes are the result of a sudden resetting of the body's thermostat. If your brain senses that your body is too hot—for any reason, including low estrogen, increased blood flow to the brain, a high ambient temperature, or even the ingestion of hot, spicy foods—it sends out a signal that your body needs to cool off. In response, your pituitary gland sends out an increased amount of luteinizing hormone (LH), which causes the blood vessels near your skin's surface to dilate to release heat through your skin. This heat-releasing action makes your skin temperature (and your body temperature) rise, followed by an increase in perspiration. The perspiration helps to cool the skin, which can result in a clammy feeling. If you've perspired heavily, you may be left damp and even chilly. Your body temperature drops and your blood vessels constrict. That's the hot flash in action.

Common Hot Flash Triggers

Other factors besides fluctuating estrogen levels can cause hot flashes or contribute to their severity. Many women find, for example, that they have hot flashes during periods of anxiety and nervousness; other studies have found that some prescription antihypertensive and antianxiety medications may also cause hot flashes. And some women report their hot flashes are more severe and last longer when they occur during hot weather or in a hot room.

How Many, How Bad, How Long?

Although many women don't seem to notice hot flashes until after menopause has occurred, many others begin having them during perimenopause, with forty-eight being an average age for the onset of hot flashes.

A number of studies have been conducted on the prevalence, frequency, and intensity of hot flashes in perimenopausal and menopausal women. In general, women who experience hot flashes start having them within at least one year before menopause and continue having them for one to six years.

The American College of Obstetricians and Gynecologists' publication *Managing Menopause* lists the findings of one study, in which 501 women were asked about the frequency and severity of their hot flashes. Of those participating in the study, 87 percent reported having one or more flashes per day; of those experiencing multiple daily hot flashes, the numbers of incidents per day ranged from five to fifty, with one-third of the women reporting more than ten. Another study reported a lower frequency of hot flashes—participants had an average of only three or four flashes a day. That study also showed that, on average, hot flashes lasted about three and one-half minutes, though some can come and go in no more than five seconds. And in nearly every study, almost three-fourths of the respondents said their hot flashes were mild, moderate, or only variably intense.

Techniques for Turning Down the Heat

If you're coping with hot flashes, you have a variety of first-defense techniques available to you that don't require any special medication or therapeutic program. Remember, the hot flash is your body's overexcitation of a normal heat-release mechanism. So, if there is less "heat" in the environment to begin with, you'll be better off. Try these simple techniques to avoid hot flashes or minimize their severity:

- **Avoid triggering foods and drinks:** Spicy foods—foods heavy in capsaicin—the heat-inducing chemical in cayenne and other hot peppers and sauces—can contribute to hot flashes. Caffeine and alcohol are also common triggers; avoid caffeinated beverages, excessive amounts of chocolate, and alcoholic beverages if you are suffering from hot flashes.

- **Drink plenty of water during the day:** It's important to drink at least thirty-two ounces daily, more if possible. Keep a glass of ice water with you during meetings and conferences and set a thermal-lined drink container of ice water on your nightstand.

- **Get at least thirty minutes of exercise every day:** Exercise, including stretching, aerobic, and weight-bearing activities, has been shown to cut down on the frequency of hot flashes and may even help limit the length and severity of hot flashes that occur. Regular exercise also promotes a general feeling of well-being that can help reduce anxiety and stress that can contribute to hot flashes.

- **Wear layers of moisture-absorbing clothing:** When a hot flash strikes, you can take off one or more layers of clothing to help cool your skin temperature quickly. Cotton fabrics in a looser size wick moisture away from the skin and into the air, so both you and your clothing can dry more quickly. Tightly woven synthetic fabrics can hold in both body heat and moisture, making the hot flash more severe and its effects more long lasting.

- **Keep your thermostat turned down:** Stay at seventy degrees or lower during the day and sixty-five degrees or lower at night. Lower temperatures can help ward off the onset of hot flashes, and you'll cool off more quickly from those that do occur when the air around you is cool. Keep a fan handy, and turn it on whenever necessary. If you suffer from night sweats, it's especially important that you keep your bedroom temperature cool; don't skimp on the air conditioning, and use a fan to keep the air moving around your room.

- **Manage stress to the best of your ability:** Avoid stress if you can, but be prepared for stressful situations you can't sidestep. Deep breathing exercises, meditation, yoga, and visualization are all helpful techniques for boosting your ability to remain calm and centered throughout your day. Massage therapy and acupressure can also help you manage your response to stress and reduce the frequency of stress-induced hot flashes.

Hormonal Treatments for Hot Flash Relief

Though medical science continues to study the connection between hormone depletion and hot flashes, hormone replacement treatment—involving estrogen and/or progesterone—is the most effective medical treatment for vasomotor symptoms known today. According to the American College of Obstetricians and Gynecologists, 80 to 90 percent of women taking prescribed estrogen find relief from hot flashes.

Prolonged Symptoms

If you suffer from severe hot flashes, it's not unusual to have feelings of nausea, headache, and weakness afterward—especially when hot flashes last for thirty or forty-five minutes. If your feelings of intense heat last for longer than an hour, you may not be experiencing symptoms of perimenopause or menopause, and you should consult your doctor or other health-care professional for a check of your thyroid function, blood sugar, and possibly other blood parameters.

Estrogen offers a number of other health benefits for women experiencing symptoms of perimenopause and menopause, including protection against osteoporosis and colorectal cancer. No other treatment for the relief of hot flashes offers the wide-ranging benefits of estrogen replacement therapy. Women using estrogen replacement for the treatment of hot flashes typically experience some relief within a few weeks of beginning treatment, though it may be a month or more before they begin to feel the maximum benefits.

Estrogen isn't recommended for women with a personal history of recently diagnosed endometrial cancer. For these women, progestins such as medroxyprogesterone or megestrol acetate have been shown to offer some relief from hot flashes.

Another hormone-based treatment for hot flashes is progesterone cream. This cream, available through prescription, is rubbed on the skin, and the progesterone is slowly absorbed into the woman's system. Do not overuse or take more of the cream than is recommended, because it can be accompanied by some negative side effects, including vaginal bleeding and PMS symptoms such as fatigue.

Only your doctor or health-care professional can help you decide whether or not hormone-based treatments are your best choice for reducing or eliminating hot flashes. If you and your health-care provider decide that hormones aren't right for you, you can choose from other treatment options, including other medications and hormone alternatives.

Quick Fix for Hot Flashes

If a hot flash strikes, you may get some quick relief by running cold water over your hands, wrists, and inner elbow. A cold cloth on your forehead or the back of your neck can help, too; if you're at home, step into a cold shower until the heat wave passes.

Nonhormonal Medications

To provide relief from hot flashes for women who cannot take estrogen, medical professionals can prescribe other medications that have been shown to offer some relief from hot flashes. The following list mentions some of these prescription medications for alleviating hot flashes:

- **Clonidine hydrochloride** reduces the responsiveness of the body's vascular system and has been used for decades in the treatment of high blood pressure. A low dose is used; it may take three to four weeks to begin to see improvement in symptoms; blood pressure must also be monitored. Clonidine has some negative side effects, however; some tests have shown that Clonidine can disrupt the sleep of some women. Other side effects reported include dizziness and dry mouth.

- **Methyldopa** is another antihypertensive (high blood pressure medication) sometimes used to relieve vasomotor symptoms. Though methyldopa has been shown to reduce the number of hot flashes women experience during the day, it can cause dry mouth, dizziness, and headache.

- **Selective serotonin reuptake inhibitors** (**SSRIs**), including paroxetine and venlafaxine, are also used to lessen vasomotor symptoms, though doctors don't commonly prescribe them for that purpose. In higher doses, these drugs are used to treat depression. Some tests have shown that relatively low doses of these drugs can reduce the frequency and severity of hot flashes by as much as 50 to 75 percent, depending upon the specific drug and dosage strategy. Side effects of these drugs include dry mouth, nausea, and anxiety.

For more information on other alternative treatments that aid in reducing symptoms of menopause, including hot flashes, see Chapter 14.

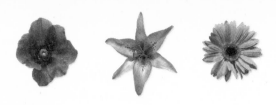

chapter six | **Understanding *Hormones* and HRT**

Hormone Replacement Therapy (HRT) has been in place for over fifty years, and though it continues to be the focus of much research and scientific debate, it remains the most studied, respected, and commonly used form of treatment for menopausal symptoms and long-term health implications of menopause. However, HRT does have risks, and it may not be right for everyone.

The Role of Hormones in Your Health

Though your body produces a number of hormones, three hormones play leading roles in your reproductive cycle—estrogen, progesterone, and androgens. All three of these hormones can be used in HRT and therefore continue to play a role in your health from puberty through your mature years.

Because hormones are such an important and widely used tool for controlling menopausal symptoms, including hot flashes, night sweats, mood swings, vaginal atrophy, and later, bone loss and deteriorating vision, they are the subject of constant, ongoing medical research. As a result, rarely a month passes that we don't hear of some new development in their use or some new question regarding their safety or efficacy. New developments emerge all the time, and new information will continue to come to light long after you read these words. In order for you to make decisions based on the best information at hand, however, you need a fundamental understanding of these basic sex hormones and how and why they're used in HRT. The sections that follow give you this basic information. Use it as a platform for a continued discussion with your doctor or other health-care provider. If your physician doesn't seem receptive to this type of interaction, now is the time to seek a second opinion.

Weigh the Pros and Cons Carefully

When considering HRT or an alternative, remember that you have more to be concerned about than the physical discomforts of hot flashes or occasional forgetfulness and mood swings. Lack of estrogen can lead to real problems such as osteoporosis and vaginal atrophy. Avoiding HRT doesn't automatically make you a "natural" woman or a stronger, more capable individual. If anything, it may leave you less capable by exposing you to multiple health problems associated with aging.

Estrogen and Its Use in HRT

Estrogen is a growth hormone that stimulates the development of adult sex organs during puberty. At puberty, estrogen promotes development of a woman's breasts and hips with what we think of as natural fat deposits and the resulting contours. Estrogen helps retain calcium in bones, a function that keeps bones strong and whole during childbearing years. It also regulates the balance of HDL and

LDL cholesterol in the bloodstream and helps lower your body's total cholesterol level. (See Chapter 8.) Estrogen aids other body functions, such as regulating blood sugar levels and emotional balance.

As you learned in Chapter 1, your body doesn't stop producing estrogen when you stop ovulating, but it produces gradually lower levels of estrogen as your ovarian function declines. Although the body continues to produce small amounts of estrogen, it's only at about 25 percent or less of its premenopause rate—levels too small to support the hormone's age-defying functions in the body.

Estrogen is used in HRT to:

- Diminish hot flashes.
- Keep the vaginal walls supple, moist, and well nourished.
- Maintain or even increase bone density.
- Improve blood cholesterol levels, stimulate blood circulation, and keep the arteries healthy, dilated, and plaque-free to help protect against heart disease.
- Help alleviate urinary tract problems and diminish stress and urge incontinence.
- Help protect cognitive function by improving circulation and increasing the flow of blood to the brain (early studies seem to indicate that it may help delay or prevent the onset of Alzheimer's disease).
- Lower the risk of age-related macular degeneration of the eye and glaucoma.
- Lower the risk of rheumatoid arthritis and Parkinson's disease.
- Reduce the risk of contracting colorectal cancer by as much as a third in most studies.

HRT and *Osteoporosis*

HRT has proven its benefit in maintaining bone health and preventing osteoporosis. Most studies show that women who use estrogen and progestin HRT compounds reduce their risk of hip fracture by 11 percent for each year of HRT treatments.

In the 1950s and 1960s, many doctors prescribed unopposed estrogen replacement, meaning that the woman received estrogen alone, without the balancing effects of the hormone progesterone, even if she had an intact uterus. But later studies revealed that estrogen given alone could result in the development of endometrial cancer (cancer of the uterine lining), so HRT today almost always involves some combination of estrogen, progesterone, and in some cases, androgens such as testosterone. If a woman has had a hysterectomy, she doesn't need to worry about endometrial cancer, so her HRT prescription should involve only estrogen—a treatment known as ERT, or Estrogen Replacement Therapy.

The Women's Health Initiative Study

Long-term studies are essential for understanding the full implications of any drug or medical treatment. The National Institutes of Health's Women's Health Initiative Study is a fifteen-year study launched in 1991 to study the most common causes of death and potential complications in postmenopausal women, including a representative sample of them who used HRT and another group taking estrogen alone.

Estrogens offer many health benefits, but these powerful hormones can have some negative effects. Estrogen can contribute to the occurrence of blood clots in the deep veins of the legs or the lungs of women who have a history of these problems. If you are considering HRT, and you don't know your family's medical history, now is the time to ask about it. If any of your immediate relatives has suffered from blood clots not caused by a predisposing risk factor such as pregnancy, prolonged bed rest, recovery from a motor vehicle accident, and so on, you need to report that information to your doctor or health-care professional. A family history of such blood clots could indicate that you, too, carry a risk for the condition; your health-care worker will use that information to determine whether he or she can recommend HRT for treatment of your menopausal symptoms.

As you progress through perimenopause, your body's hormonal changes take place over a period of months or years, giving your system time to adjust to gradually declining hormone levels. If you go through an induced menopause, your menopause will be immediate and, very likely, dramatic in its physical impact and symptoms. In those cases, your doctor or health-care provider is likely to recommend some form of estrogen replacement to help your body through the transition.

Progesterone and Its Use in HRT

Normally, your ovaries produce progesterone in the process of ovulation, so most women in their reproductive years that report having regular menstrual cycles would be expected to have normal progesterone levels. Progesterone has a counterbalancing, stabilizing impact on tissue growth; progesterone helps keep the growth of your uterine lining (endometrium) in check, for example, thereby keeping your cycles regular and predictable. In your childbearing years, progesterone also promotes the development of nutrients in the uterus, breasts, and fallopian tubes to prepare your body for a possible pregnancy.

Your progesterone levels drop dramatically when you stop ovulating.

Because a woman's body produces the majority of its progesterone during the second half of the ovulatory cycle, if you don't ovulate, your progesterone supply falls. Failure to ovulate is probably the first and most common explanation for irregular cycles that begin in perimenopause (although some women do experience anovulatory cycles earlier in life). Because progesterone's most important effect in your body is its estrogen-balancing capabilities, most HRT prescriptions for women who still have a uterus include some type of progestin, a pharmaceutically prepared form of the naturally occurring hormone progesterone.

Progestin serves several important purposes in HRT. It helps to mediate the growth-stimulating functions of estrogen, so it reduces the risk of endometrial cancer for women who still have their uterus. In spite of its critical importance for balancing the effects of estrogen in HRT, however, progestin has its drawbacks. Some women experience breast tenderness and water retention when taking progestin with estrogen in an HRT regimen. Other women find that some forms of progestin aggravate mood swings. And many forms of progestin can diminish the heart-healthy effects of estrogen, which is why doctors don't include progestin therapy in HRT if a woman has had a hysterectomy.

For these reasons, doctors and health-care providers monitor HRT patients carefully to determine which progestin type and delivery technique works best for each individual. If you have a medical history of high cholesterol or high cholesterol fractions, such as LDL (the "bad" cholesterol) or triglycerides, discuss it with your doctor before deciding on an HRT prescription.

A number of different types of progestins are available, including:

- Medroxyprogesterone acetate (MPA), used in brand names such as Provera, Cycrin, and found in estrogen combination compounds such as PremPro and PremPhase.

- Norethindrone or other 19-nortestosterone derivatives in estrogen/progestin combinations such as CombiPatch and FemHRT.
- Micronized oral progesterone, marketed as Prometrium.
- Norgestimate, as found in Prefest.

Progestin can be taken continuously or cyclically ten to fourteen days of every month or every other month. Progestins given in a cyclic fashion usually produce a predictable menstrual period; progestins given in the same dose on a daily basis are designed to make most women amenorrheic, or period-free, after one year of therapy or sooner.

Androgens and Their Use in HRT

Androgens are male hormones (the most common of which is testosterone), normally produced in small quantities by the ovaries and adrenal glands, with the greatest quantities occurring at the midpoint of a woman's cycle. Androgens contribute to bone density (though not as dramatically as do estrogens), and some studies show that they might promote a healthy libido by fostering a desire for sex. Androgen production also drops dramatically when ovarian function decreases around the time of menopause. The decrease is even more dramatic if a woman undergoes a surgical menopause. If women have severe menopausal symptoms such as intermittent hot flashes or a greatly reduced sex drive, despite a trial of traditional HRT, their health-care providers may recommend an HRT regimen that includes androgens.

HRT and *Symptoms*

Irregular bleeding or spotting is the most common complaint of women who have recently begun HRT, while others report breast tenderness and water retention. And, while some women say HRT contributes to migraines, others say it actually helps ameliorate migraine problems they've experienced for years. Keep a symptom calendar that includes your prescription medications and when you take them.

The use of androgens to combat menopausal symptoms is relatively new. Some studies have shown that androgen in combination with estrogen not only slows bone loss but also may help promote the growth of new bone. Some experts believe androgens can help alleviate other menopausal symptoms such as hot flashes and vaginal dryness, at least in some people. Androgens carry some negative risks, of course; studies do show that androgens can have a negative effect on blood cholesterol levels (raising LDL and decreasing HDL, instead of the opposite), and a few patients who take androgens can experience unwanted side effects, such as the growth of excess facial hair, acne, or oiliness of the skin. In general, androgens are added to an HRT regimen only if libido or hot flashes are not improved on standard HRT dosages.

The Facts about HRT

Menopausal and postmenopausal women have a variety of alternatives for protecting their health and diminishing menopausal symptoms. The most popular and proven of these is hormone replacement therapy. However, many women are reluctant to begin HRT, and many women who start HRT discontinue it within six months. HRT isn't for everyone. Your family or personal medical history may make you a poor candidate for hormone replacement therapy. Or you may choose to use other methods for maintaining your health and alleviating menopausal symptoms. However, your choice should be based on fact—not unnecessary fears or unfounded beliefs about the safety or beneficial impact of this treatment option. This section presents those facts.

Unfortunately, much of the information proffered to the public about HRT is biased or misleading—based on improperly or incompletely designed and performed studies. Some media seem dedicated to promoting only controversial or negative findings regarding health-care issues and the medical establishment, in order to fan the public's fear (and boost ratings). Your trained, licensed health-care provider is your first and best source of complete information and advice about HRT, how it works, and what risks and benefits it offers you. Subspecialists are a good option for a second opinion or complicated cases.

Online Information about Prescription Drugs

If you have access to the Internet, you can turn to the National Institutes of Health's National Medical Library for authoritative information about most drugs prescribed today. Use the Library's topic list, drug information, and dictionaries to find out how any drug works, how it's prescribed, and its potential side effects and interactions. Find the library at *www.nlm.nih.gov* (click on MEDLINEplus).

Who Uses HRT?

Hormone replacement therapy is used by fewer than half of all menopausal women in the United States. The reasons for using—or not using—HRT vary from individual to individual, but many women who aren't on HRT have yet to make a decision regarding its use. The decision to follow an HRT regimen is an important one for any woman; as soon as your ovarian function diminishes, your hormone levels plummet. Whatever technique you use to minimize postmenopausal bone loss, heart disease, memory function loss, and other effects of diminished hormones, you need to begin it before those losses build. Here's what we know about the women who choose HRT and why they choose it:

- Most surveys indicate that the main reason women between the ages of fifty and fifty-five choose to begin HRT is for the relief of hot flashes and other vasomotor symptoms. Women who begin HRT at age sixty-five and older are more likely to be concerned with preventing or postponing the onset of osteoporosis.
- Almost 40 percent of menopausal women turn to HRT for the relief of night sweats and vaginal dryness—in addition to hot flashes.
- Nearly 50 percent of women currently using HRT have undergone a hysterectomy. In those cases, over 35 percent of current HRT users and over 40 percent of past users turned to HRT as a result of surgically induced menopause. Understandably, women who no longer have a uterus have little concern over the most common side effect, irregular vaginal bleeding; and these women are most likely to have experienced sudden, severe hot flashes.

The Risks of HRT

If you read the newspaper, listen to the evening news, or pick up any women's magazine, you're likely to read or hear about ongoing research into the risks and benefits of HRT almost daily. Because HRT has been under study for so long, some reports about its potential risks are inevitable, but further study is needed to understand fully its long-term effects. Any medication carries certain risks. Here are the HRT risks most women must consider:

Breast cancer: A small number of recent studies suggest that long-term (more than five years) use of HRT may result in a small but increased risk of breast cancer. Though this risk appears to be small, most health-care professionals advise women who have a personal history of breast cancer against using HRT for at least the first five years following their diagnoses. Regardless of their use of HRT or family history, all menopausal women should get regular mammograms, conduct monthly breast self-exams, and visit their physician annually.

Endometrial cancer: If you still have your uterus, you shouldn't take unopposed estrogen (estrogen without progesterone) for the sole purpose of relief of menopausal symptoms because unopposed estrogen can increase your risk of developing endometrial cancer. HRT regimens that balance estrogen with progestin eliminate this risk, however, and do in fact reduce the risk of endometrial cancer even further compared to women who take no hormone supplements at all. If you have been treated successfully for early (Stage I through III) endometrial cancer, with a total hysterectomy, your doctor may recommend an ERT regimen for you after a certain disease-free interval, to insure there is no evidence of recurrence of the cancer, usually after three to five years.

Blood clots: If you have ever developed blood clots in the deep veins of your legs or in your lungs or eyes, you may be susceptible to redeveloping them if you use HRT. High levels of estrogen can contribute to this condition, so your health-care professional will want to test your current blood hormone levels and review your history to see if you are a good candidate for HRT. Low-dose estrogen treatments may not complicate your risks for recurring blood clots, and your doctor may recommend that HRT option. Your doctor can order special blood tests that check for clotting difficulties, if your family or personal medical history raises any question about an inherited susceptibility.

Liver disease: If you have active liver disease or if your liver's function has become seriously impaired through illness or injury, you aren't a good candidate for HRT. Your liver is the organ that metabolizes (breaks down) the estrogen in your circulatory system. If your liver isn't functioning properly, your body won't be able to metabolize the estrogen component of HRT. If your liver disease is resolved, however, the potential for an increased risk may have passed. Your doctor or health-care professional can advise you whether your liver function (usually based on blood tests for liver enzymes) makes you a suitable candidate for HRT.

The increased risk of breast cancer is slight; most studies indicate that among women who took estrogen for five years, HRT contributed to only one additional case of breast cancer in every 1,000 women. The overall risk of breast cancer for women age sixty to sixty-five who aren't taking estrogen is low—about 350 of every 100,000 women on average. That number rises to 400 of every 100,000 for women of the same age who take estrogen. Regular mammograms are the key to proper monitoring.

Other Factors

Other factors may discourage women from using HRT. Many women haven't the funds for ongoing medical therapy and are uninsured or underinsured and therefore can't afford it. These women face multiple challenges in finding affordable alternatives to HRT, since many insurance programs refuse to cover certain alternative treatments. Additionally, some women may choose to avoid medical treatment as a result of religious or philosophical beliefs. Hopefully, these women have not been misinformed or misled by the media or well-meaning, but less-informed relatives and friends.

HRT may not play as beneficial a role in protecting women against heart disease as was once thought. Results of the Women's Health Initiative study, initially released in July 2002, revealed a slight increase in nonfatal heart attack, stroke, and pulmonary embolus in women taking HRT, as compared to women taking placebo alone.

When the final, complete results of the long-term Women's Health Initiative are published (in 2005), the medical and scientific communities will have a clearer understanding of the long-term benefits and risks of HRT, although many epidemiologists think that the study is raising more questions than it is answering. Until then, discuss all of your options, concerns, and questions with your health-care provider, and make an informed decision. Don't let unspecified fears or suspicions stop you in your tracks when you're preparing a health plan for this important phase of your adult life.

HRT Options

Because HRT is such a widely used and studied method of treatment, a number of different HRT compounds and delivery methods have developed over the years. You and your doctor can determine the form that's best for you, but here are some of the most popular options:

- **Pills** can offer estrogen or estrogen/progestin combinations that are taken continuously or cyclically.
- **Patches** can deliver a steady dose of estrogen or estrogen/progestin combinations every day of the month. You change the patch every three to seven days, and you can and should wear them when swimming or showering. (Don't remove a partially used patch and try to reuse it, for example, after swimming.)
- **Flexible vaginal rings** deliver estrogen in steady doses to women

who suffer from vaginal dryness. Certain forms are available that make estrogen replacement safe even for breast cancer patients, because the estrogen works locally (in the vagina) and is not absorbed into the bloodstream (which could increase the potential for the recurrence of the cancer).

- **Creams** that provide topical estrogen for women who suffer from vaginal dryness are available. These creams are inserted directly into the vagina. Progesterone gels and creams can be applied directly on the skin, such as the skin of the abdomen or the arm. Again, your health-care provider can advise you on the proper dose and delivery mechanism for these (and all) forms of HRT. Be careful: Some progesterone creams are not approved or regulated by the FDA and, as such, may not deliver a pharmaceutical dose of sufficient progesterone to protect the endometrium from developing endometrial hyperplasia.

A new option, called low-dose HRT, has shown promising results in recent studies. The reduced levels of hormones are effective in reducing symptoms and cause very little irregular vaginal bleeding—one of the primary objections many women express to traditional HRT. The protection against osteoporosis conferred by the lower dose is nearly the same as that seen with the standard dose, and the improvement in hot flashes is nearly as successful.

Consult with Your Doctor Before Using Plant Estrogens

If you have your uterus, your health-care professional won't prescribe unopposed estrogen for treatment of menopausal symptoms. Be aware, however, that if you self-medicate with plant estrogens (phytoestrogens) from soy foods or supplements, you may be giving your body unopposed estrogens. Talk to your health-care provider about any and all supplements and vitamins you take on a regular basis.

It is anticipated that the future trend in HRT will be toward the use of the lowest possible doses that can treat vasomotor symptoms and still reduce a woman's risk for bone fractures. Talk with your doctor or health-care provider for more details.

"Designer" Estrogens

In the past several years, a number of artificial estrogens have been developed to provide some of the benefits of estrogen replacement therapy while avoiding some of the risks for women who aren't good candidates for HRT. These compounds work as estrogen receptor "foolers": They act like estrogens in some of the body's tissues, but they don't act like estrogens with others. These "designer estrogens" are more correctly referred to as selective estrogen receptor modulators or SERMs. SERMs are useful for combating bone loss in postmenopausal patients who can't or choose not to use HRT, but who are still at risk of developing osteoporosis. Following are the most common SERMs in use today.

- **Tamoxifen** (sold under the brand name Nolvadex) has been in use for some years to help reduce the potential for recurrence of estrogen-dependent breast cancer in women with a history of that disease. Ongoing studies of Tamoxifen indicate it isn't an "ideal answer" for postmenopausal women. Although it maintains bone density, it has been linked to an increased risk of endometrial polyps, blood clots, and possibly precancerous endometrial hyperplasia.

- **Raloxifene** was approved by the FDA in 1997 for use in the prevention of osteoporosis and is marketed under the brand name Evista. Raloxifene has been found to maintain a certain amount of bone density, at least in some patients, without increasing the risk of breast or uterine cancer. Because it doesn't appear to have any adverse effects on the endometrium, women who still have their uterus don't need to take progestin or progesterone when on Raloxifene. However, Raloxifene seems to be only about half as effective as estrogen at increasing bone density. Raloxifene also appears to reduce LDL cholesterol; it has been shown to do so without increasing "good" HDL cholesterol the way estrogen does. The risk of blood clots with Raloxifene seems to be similar to that of estrogen, and Raloxifene has shown no beneficial effect in reducing hot flashes. It actually increases hot flashes in some patients.

Watch for New SERMs

Though SERMs show great promise for the development of post-menopausal treatment without the risks of traditional hormones, long-term studies are still in progress. Newer SERMs with fewer side effects are in development.

Weighing Risks and Benefits

When you meet with your health-care professional to discuss treatment options, be sure to ask about the following tests and discuss risk factors.

- Talk to your doctor about your personal and family history of osteoporosis, heart disease, breast cancer, blood clots, colon cancer, and liver disease.

- Ask about a bone density test to determine the current state of your bone health. A heel or peripheral bone density test may give you all the information you need and is cheaper and quicker to perform than some more detailed bone examinations. It is especially appropriate the first time you are screened for osteoporosis.
- Request a fasting blood test called a "lipid" or "coronary profile" to find out your levels of total cholesterol, HDL, LDL, and triglycerides to determine your cardiac disease risk.
- Ask your doctor about the usefulness of blood tests to determine your current blood hormone levels or how close you are to menopause. An FSH blood test is considered most useful.

Irregular Bleeding

More than half of the women who experience irregular spotting or bleeding after beginning an HRT regimen that includes progestin stop bleeding completely after six months; 80 percent stop bleeding within a year. Continued bleeding (after one year) may indicate an anatomical, most likely preexisting problem with the lining of the uterus rather than a side effect of HRT. (See "Fibroids, Polyps, and Other Sources of Heavy or Irregular Bleeding" in Chapter 7.)

- Keep your menstrual calendar and menopausal symptom diary (see Chapter 3) and take it with you to your doctor's appointments in order to discuss the symptoms you've been having and their severity, so you know what kind of symptom relief you need most.
- Ask your doctor or health-care professional about alternatives to HRT, their benefits, and their drawbacks.
- Get regular medical checkups. Your doctor will recommend annual or semi-annual examinations to monitor the progress of

your HRT program. During the annual exam, your health-care provider will check your breasts for lumps; do a pelvic exam to evaluate your uterus, cervix, vagina, and ovaries; and check your blood pressure. Don't skip these appointments; they're an important part of your HRT program.

• Ask about screening for colon cancer. Colonoscopy is recommended for everyone at age 50 and earlier for patients with a positive family history of colon cancer or its precursors.

HRT Is Just Part of a Healthy Menopause Plan

Hormone replacement therapy offers an enormous number of benefits for women in menopause and postmenopause. But remember, lifestyle and behavioral changes are an important part of a complete plan for a healthy life—before, during, and after the onset of menopause. No pill, patch, or cream will keep you healthy if you live an unhealthy lifestyle. As you grow older, your health maintenance becomes more critical—and more demanding. So even if you adopt a full program of HRT—or use any HRT alternative—you need to follow the other guidelines discussed in this book to maintain your good health.

Follow Your HRT Program Faithfully

Remember to follow your HRT program exactly as prescribed. Many people forget their schedule and miss doses. Use whatever reminder mechanism works for you—a weekly pill container, a marked calendar, notes on your mirror, or other device. If you can't find a reminder that works, ask your health-care professional for advice. But don't miss doses or double-up just out of curiosity!

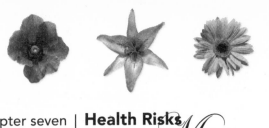

chapter seven | **Health Risks
Related to Menopause**

Many women are healthier than they've ever been as they approach midlife. Nevertheless, a well-thought-out approach to health management and maintenance is smart at any age, and it becomes more important as each year passes. Don't think of your health-care efforts as part of entering old age; think of them as a simple, basic plan to stay young and healthy.

For women, the physical effects of an aging reproductive system can present some special health risks. Estrogen provides women with a natural protection against certain diseases. In perimenopause, because a woman's body produces less estrogen, she becomes more vulnerable to certain health risks. Many physical symptoms that might be attributed to the first pangs of aging might actually be the warning signals of serious health problems in the making. A good health-care regimen at age forty can lay the groundwork for a healthy passage through ages fifty, sixty, seventy, eighty, and beyond.

The following sections of this chapter look at some of the most common age-related health factors that deserve your attention as you approach menopause. (Osteoporosis and heart disease—two of the most important health risks to consider—are covered separately in subsequent chapters.) When you understand the types of health risks and issues you may face, you can begin creating your midlife health-management strategy.

Cancer Risks

Though heart disease is a more common disease among American women, cancer is one of the most feared. Cancer is the second leading cause of death in the United States; nearly four of every ten Americans will have some kind of cancer at some point during their lives, and nearly 80 percent of those diagnosed with cancer are age fifty-five or older. One-third of all women in the United States will develop cancer during their lifetimes, so as you approach menopause, it's important that you understand which cancers have age-related risk factors for women.

Cancer is a family of diseases, all of which occur when cell growth becomes abnormal and goes out of control in some part of the body. Cancer has been widely studied, but its causes are complex and still not fully understood. Contributing factors include environmental pollutants, heredity, occupation, nutrition, and lifestyle. At times, there is no medical explanation for why a certain type of cancer develops in a previously healthy person. Different cancers produce different illnesses, each with its own symptoms, causes, and risk factors. The following sections discuss some of the most common cancers women face as they move into middle age. The object of this information isn't to alarm you. Rather, this brief overview will alert you to the risks your health-management plan should monitor.

#1 Cancer Threat for Women: Lung Cancer

Lung cancer is the leading cause of cancer death for women in the United States, and tobacco smoke is the leading cause of lung cancer. The

American Lung Association reports that nearly 68,000 women died in the United States from lung cancer in 2000, as opposed to 41,000 who died from breast cancer. Most women are diagnosed with lung cancer at age fifty—right around the time they hit menopause, often after thirty-five or more years of tobacco smoke exposure. Women are twice as likely as men to contract cancer from tobacco smoke, and the vast majority of nonsmokers who contract lung cancer are women.

If you're approaching menopause, the time is right for you to quit smoking—now. Smoking increases your chances of contracting cervical cancer, emphysema, and other life-threatening chronic lung conditions. The effects of smoking will complicate any illness you contract.

Don't Be Afraid to Quit Smoking

Since 1950, lung cancer deaths in women in the United States have increased by a startling 600 percent. Every woman smoker knows she should quit, but many fear weight gain, anxiety, and unquenchable cravings during withdrawal. Don't be afraid; you have more options for quitting now than ever before, including patches, gum, medications, and hypnosis. Do whatever it takes to quit now.

Quitting smoking can give you health benefits right away. According to the American Cancer Society (ACS), within twenty minutes after you quit, your body starts regenerating and your blood pressure begins to return to normal. Within eight hours, the carbon monoxide level in your blood drops to normal. Twenty-four hours after you quit, your chance of heart attack begins to decrease. One to nine months later, you should lose that smoker's cough and the sinus congestion, fatigue, and shortness of breath smokers suffer. Within ten years of quitting, you will have cut your risk of lung-cancer death in half; after fifteen years, your chance of contracting coronary heart disease is the same as that of a nonsmoker.

#2 Cancer Threat for Women: Breast Cancer

Breast cancer is the second most common form of cancer contracted by women today, and advancing age appears to be a major risk factor in its development. Nearly 80 percent of all breast cancers are found in women over fifty, and the incidence of diagnosis and fatality both seem to increase with age. The American Cancer Society (ACS) reports that 163 per 100,000 women in the United States in their forties are diagnosed with breast cancer each year, and 29 die of it; 374 per 100,000 women in their sixties will be diagnosed, and 90 of those will die from the disease. Age isn't the sole risk factor; heredity, lifestyle, family health history, and personal health history, including early onset of menstruation (before age twelve) and late menopause (after fifty-five), all can have an impact on your likelihood of developing breast cancer.

If your mother, sister, or daughter has had breast cancer, your risks of contracting it go up two to three times (depending on how many of these first-degree relatives are involved). And, if you've had breast cancer before, you have a higher risk of developing it again. If you've never had a child or had your first child after age thirty, your risk goes up as well. But what about risk factors that you can change? The American Cancer Society lists the following risk factors for breast cancer that are specifically linked to lifestyle choices:

Hormone replacement therapy (HRT): Most large studies and most world experts agree that long-term use of estrogen alone after menopause (ERT) does not increase your risk of breast cancer. However, according to the ACS, a very few studies suggest that long-term use (ten or more years) of estrogen and progesterone together, or HRT, may result in a slight increase in risk. The connection between breast cancer and HRT is still the subject of ongoing research. Some medical professionals suspect that women who take estrogen are more likely to do breast self-exams, see their physicians regularly, and have mammograms. These women are more likely to have their cancers diagnosed at an early stage, usually before they can even be palpated by the physician or on a breast self-exam, so these tiny cancers can be cured with conservative surgery such as lumpectomy. These women also live longer than their counterparts who take no hormones, presumably due to their regular medical checkups and the protective effect of estrogen on the heart.

Alcohol: Women who have one alcoholic drink a day have a slightly increased risk of contracting breast cancer; two to five drinks daily can up your risk to one and one-half times that of nondrinkers.

Diet: The connection between obesity and breast cancer risk is still being studied, but research indicates that after menopause, your risk of contracting breast cancer is greater if you are overweight. How much of this risk is linked to your body fat versus specific dietary fat content is still under debate. Another issue may be that more breast tissue (obese women tend to have bigger breasts) makes it harder to find an early, small cancerous lump, both on exam and on mammogram.

Exercise: Early findings reported by the ACS seem to indicate that even moderate physical activity can lower breast cancer risk. Maintaining good overall physical condition certainly improves your chances of having fewer complications related to medical and surgical treatment for any disease—including breast cancer.

Survival rates for breast cancer are highest when the cancer is detected early. The five-year survival rate (your chance of being alive five years after being diagnosed with cancer) is 96 percent for women whose cancer is caught at an early stage. Early detection helps keep the surgery or other treatment that follows diagnosis as noninvasive and conservative as is possible.

Breast Self-Exams

Breast self-exams are your first line of defense against breast cancer. Ask your health-care provider to demonstrate how to check your breasts for lumps or growths or visit *www.cancer.org* for a good, visual guide to this procedure. Self-exams must be accompanied by annual mammograms after age forty, especially when you have a positive family history.

Endometrial Cancer

In the United States, cancer of the endometrium—the lining of the uterus—is the most common cancer of the female reproductive organs. The ACS expected that over 36,000 new cases of endometrial cancer would be diagnosed in the United States during 2001; this cancer has a five-year survival rate of about 84 percent.

Your risk of developing endometrial cancer increases as you age. The average age of diagnosis for this cancer is sixty, and 95 percent of all endometrial cancer occurs in women age forty or older.

A number of risk factors can contribute to the development of endometrial cancer:

Total number of years of menstruation: Your body's total lifetime exposure to estrogen, without the balancing hormone progesterone, can have an impact on your likelihood of developing endometrial cancer. If you began having periods at a young age, continued having periods past age fifty, and have had few or no children (which gives your body a break from constant estrogen production), your ovaries have been producing estrogen for a greater number of years than the average woman. The more estrogen (and less progesterone) your body has experienced over the years, the higher your risk of developing endometrial cancer.

Obesity: Depending upon how obese you are, your excess body fat can increase your chances of developing endometrial cancer two to five times. Body fat can convert other hormones into estrogen, and having excess body fat contributes to a woman's estrogen levels—and risks of developing this cancer. Diets high in animal fats also may contribute to this risk factor, as can diabetes—a disease common among obese women. Women who are overweight are also more likely to have abnormal menstrual periods because their ovaries fail to ovulate—thus not producing enough progesterone in relation to their estrogen.

Estrogen replacement therapy (ERT): ERT—hormone therapy that doesn't include progesterone—can increase a woman's chance of developing endometrial cancer. Though years ago doctors used to prescribe ERT for relief from hot flashes, osteoporosis, and heart disease, today doctors almost exclusively combine estrogen with progesterone in HRT, which eliminates the increased risk of endometrial cancer. Of course, if you have had a hysterectomy, you do not need a prescription for progesterone added to your estrogen, since your risk of endometrial cancer is zero.

If endometrial cancer is diagnosed early, the survival rate is excellent. Precancerous changes, such as endometrial hyperplasia, often become known through unusual spotting or bleeding. Often, these symptoms are apparent for years before actual cancer develops. Sometimes women have had irregular periods for their entire lives and forget to report this to their health-care practitioner. Besides, when you're entering menopause, irregular bleeding and spotting aren't supposed to be unusual occurrences at all, so how do you know when to worry that your irregularity is signaling endometrial cancer?

Unfortunately, Pap smears—which are great at detecting cervical cancer—don't reveal endometrial cancer. And many women assume that a normal Pap smear is an assurance of perfect gynecologic health. The best way to stay on top of this and other risks is to provide your health-caregiver with a complete family and personal health history so he or she can best monitor your health. If you suffer from unusual bleeding that lasts more than two weeks, consult your doctor right away—no matter what your medical history. A simple office test called an endometrial biopsy can determine whether or not your symptoms point to endometrial cancer or some other cause.

Ovarian Cancer

One in fifty-seven women will develop ovarian cancer over the course of her life; it's the fourth leading cause of cancer deaths in women in the United States. Every year, U.S. doctors diagnose over 23,000 cases of this cancer, and more than 14,000 women die from it. Ovarian cancer occurs most often in women who are approaching the age of menopause. This cancer is a silent killer—symptoms can be mild, vague, and similar to those of many other conditions and diseases. If detected early, while still in the ovary (called Stage I), this cancer is curable about 90 percent of the time. But if the cancer spreads to the pelvis or beyond (Stage III or IV), which is when it is most commonly diagnosed, the five-year survival rate drops dramatically. Taking all stages into consideration, this cancer's overall five-year survival rate is somewhere around 40 percent.

Sadly, early ovarian cancer has few symptoms, so it makes sense to know your risk factors and your family history.

- A family history of ovarian, breast, colon, rectal, endometrial, or pancreatic cancer increases a woman's risks considerably. The severity of increased risk is higher if there has been one of these cancers in a first-degree relative, such as a mother, sister, or daughter.
- A woman's risk of developing ovarian cancer also rises with the total number of times she has ovulated; again, exposure to estrogen has an impact on the woman's overall risks. In other words, not having had any children or not taking the birth control pill at any point in your life means your ovaries have been working overtime, compared to women in the average population.

Symptoms of ovarian cancer are vague, especially in the early stage, but can include pain, pressure, or swelling in your abdomen; gas, nausea, and indigestion; unexplained changes in your bowel movements; changes in your weight; fatigue; or pain during intercourse. If you exhibit any of these symptoms, talk to your doctor. He or she can perform a sonogram (ultrasound examination of the pelvis) to determine if your ovaries have any abnormalities. In addition, your health-care provider may choose to obtain a blood test called CA-125 to check for a certain protein that can point to the presence of ovarian tumors. It is not a perfect test. An elevated result does not always mean ovarian cancer—it can point to liver problems, colon conditions such as diverticulitis, and other illnesses. Inaccurate results with this blood test (a false-positive) are highest in premenopausal women, so check with your doctor about the usefulness of taking the test and whether it's covered by your insurance.

Similar Cancer Risk Factors

If you have had breast or ovarian cancer, you may have an increased risk for developing endometrial cancer. Some of the same risk factors contribute to all of these forms of cancer, so with the diagnosis of one, your physician will also monitor you closely for these other cancer types.

Of course, your health-care provider physically palpates your ovaries every year during your pelvic examination to detect any changes in their size or shape. In most cases, a combination of symptoms and physical examination findings lead to a formal diagnostic series of tests for ovarian cancer. That's why it's critical to report unusual physical symptoms or changes in your normal menstrual cycle to your health-care provider.

Fibroids, Polyps, and Other Sources of Heavy or Irregular Bleeding

Irregular bleeding isn't uncommon during perimenopause. Because you ovulate less frequently, your body's estrogen levels often are unchecked by progesterone. As a result, your uterine lining can develop abnormal cell changes that lead to unusually heavy bleeding or spotting.

Fibroids are benign growths of muscle tissue that develop within the wall of the uterus, on the uterine lining, or on the outside of the uterus. Two out of five women in their forties can expect to develop these growths.

Fibroids within the uterine lining can cause abnormal bleeding because of the way they distort the lining and prevent it from shedding normally. Fibroids can sometimes become quite large. Their size alone can cause problems, such as pelvic discomfort, bloating, or pain during intercourse. If you have unusually heavy or midcycle bleeding, your doctor probably will check for fibroids.

Fibroids usually shrink after menopause. As a result, your doctor may or may not choose to treat them with surgery or drugs, depending upon the severity of your symptoms. Conservative treatment options are now also available, usually done as outpatient surgery—a hysteroscopy. In this sophisticated dilation and curettage (D and C) procedure, a small (⅛-inch) camera lens and instrument port is inserted into the cervix to locate the fibroids or polyps and remove them.

Polyps are smaller benign growths on the lining of the uterus. Polyps bleed, just like fibroids, but because they typically are small, they're unlikely to cause the amount of blood loss associated with fibroids. When a health-care provider diagnoses polyps (usually through an ultrasound test or a biopsy sample), he or she can remove them through a simple outpatient procedure that usually involves a hysteroscopy similar to that used to remove fibroids.

A common cause of abnormal bleeding is a precancerous condition of the lining of the uterus—endometrial hyperplasia. This excessive growth of the uterine lining can result from relatively low levels of progesterone. If diagnosed when still in its early stages, it can be treated medically. Untreated endometrial hyperplasia can develop into endometrial cancer.

Urinary Tract Disorders and Yeast Infections

During perimenopause, about 40 percent of women experience some form of urogenital changes—changes to the vagina, genitals, and urinary tract. The most common of these changes result from vaginal atrophy. Thin, inelastic vaginal tissue is more easily irritated and broken and therefore more prone to infections such as vaginitis, yeast infections, and urinary tract infections (UTIs). The severity of these disorders ranges from mildly irritating to very painful.

Most women have experienced some type of vaginitis (a swollen, red, irritated vaginal area) at some point in life. These infections include bacterial vaginosis, yeast infections, and trichomoniasis. During perimenopause, fluctuating hormone levels can contribute to the frequency and severity of these infections. Bacteria in the vagina, obesity, diabetes, and antibiotics are other contributors. The symptoms of these vaginal infections include burning and itching in the vaginal area and a discharge.

If you've had yeast infections before and are relatively certain that you're suffering from this type of infection, you can use over-the-counter creams and other treatments. But if you experience new or unusual symptoms or the symptoms continue or recur (especially after using an over-the-counter medication), see your physician for a full diagnosis and treatment. And although you can't prevent all vaginal infections, here are some ways to avoid them:

- Don't wear tight clothes (such as jeans) that block air circulation to your lower body, and don't wear underpants to bed at night.
- Wear underwear and pantyhose with cotton crotches.
- Be clean, clean, clean; wash your genital area thoroughly, front to back, every day, but . . .
- Stay away from heavily perfumed and deodorizing soaps, douches, sprays, tampons, and pads, and use white unscented toilet paper. Perfumes and deodorant chemicals can dry out your skin and upset the normal acid-base levels in your vagina, which can lead to infections.

Fewer layers of clothing are better than too many (though layering the clothes on your upper body is a good idea when you suffer from hot flashes); looser is better than too tight; and natural fabrics such as cotton are better than spandex and other "unbreathable" blends. After exercising, swimming, or otherwise working up a sweat, change out of sweaty clothes and get into something clean and dry.

Urinary tract infections (UTIs) are common in women of all ages, but can be particularly persistent following menopause. The lactobacilli organisms that help fight off bacterial infections in the vagina decline after menopause. UTIs, including cystitis and urethritis, are caused by bacteria (usually from skin around the anus) traveling through the urethra and reaching the bladder or even the kidneys. These bacteria trigger infections that result in symptoms such as pain or burning during urination; sudden, strong, and frequent urges to urinate; fever and chills; and even pain in your back, side, or abdomen.

Report Variations in Your Periods

The least common cause of irregular bleeding is cancer. But, because endometrial cancer can masquerade as common irregular or heavy menstrual bleeding, it's important to talk to your doctor when your periods become too heavy, too frequent, or vary noticeably from your own personal norm.

Bacteria from the bladder can rise to the kidneys. If you have painful urination, accompanied by pain in your back and fever, you may have a kidney infection. If you have painful and frequent urination, you may have a bladder infection (sometimes called cystitis). Kidney infections can result in chronic and even life-threatening consequences and bladder infections can also grow worse if untreated; contact your doctor if you experience any of these symptoms.

Sometimes more than one course of antibiotics or a different type of antibiotic is necessary to completely eradicate the bacteria.

If recurrent UTIs or symptoms that resemble UTIs become a problem for you, your doctor or health-care provider might also recommend estrogen cream or HRT to help rejuvenate your vaginal tissue. The estrogen helps increase the blood circulation to this area and restores natural secretions, thus making the entire vagina less susceptible to trauma. But you might be able to avoid some of these infections or discomforts through some simple, healthy habits:

- Wipe from front to back, so you don't push bacteria from your anus over your vaginal tissue and urethra.
- Drink lots of fluids (water is best) and urinate frequently to keep your urethra (the opening to the bladder) flushed out.
- Keep your vaginal area clean and chemical-free; wash your genital area daily and avoid any feminine hygiene products that contain additional chemicals.
- Practice clean, safe sex, and always urinate after sex to flush bacteria from your urethra. It's a good idea for both partners to wash hands and genitals before having sex.
- Use a water-based lubricant (rather than an oil-based product such as petroleum jelly) to reduce friction during intercourse.

Assessing Your Health History

Knowing your family's medical history is one of the best tools you have for predicting your future health. Your doctor or health-care provider will want and need to know this information in order to monitor your health, prescribe appropriate treatment, and recommend appropriate preventative measures. If you aren't well versed in the medical history of your parents, grandparents, and siblings, talk to your family members ahead of time to gather this information. If members of your immediate family died at an early age from medical conditions, ask other family members about those individuals' lifestyles and living conditions. The more you—and your doctor—know about the health problems that your relatives have experienced, the better able you'll be to develop a lifestyle and health maintenance plan to help protect you from inherited risks.

Don't forget your own medical history. Your doctor or healthcare professional will want to know about what illnesses, diseases, surgeries, hospitalizations, and other health issues you've experienced.

Just remember that medical science can't do it all. You have to take responsibility for living healthfully. This includes eating healthfully, drinking lots of water, quitting smoking, giving yourself monthly breast exams, using condoms and proper contraception if you're sexually active, and reducing your stress levels.

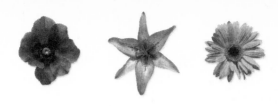

chapter eight | **What You Should Know about Heart Disease**

The umbrella term "heart disease" covers a wide range of diseases, illnesses, and events that impact the heart and circulatory system—known as cardiovascular diseases. High blood pressure and coronary artery disease that can lead to stroke, heart attacks, and early death are some of the most common forms of heart disease for both men and women. The problems that contribute to heart disease can grow silently over a number of years. Even the first signs of serious heart illness, such as a heart attack or stroke, can be attributed to other causes and therefore go unrecognized.

Heart disease is the number-one killer of women over fifty in America today: According to the American Heart Association, one out of two women will die of cardiovascular disease, and the number of women who die of heart disease has reached over 500,000 a year. It's true that prior to menopause women suffer fewer effects of heart disease and stroke than men. But as women age, their risk of heart disease increases dramatically. More than half of all stroke deaths occur in women.

Some studies indicate that a woman's natural estrogen loss due to aging may contribute to certain types of heart disease. Estrogen can help control the body's blood cholesterol levels, and it keeps a woman's total cholesterol low before menopause, with low levels of LDL (low-density lipoproteins or "bad" cholesterol) and high levels of "good" cholesterol, HDL (high-density lipoproteins). These fractions are reversed after menopause and are thought to be serious contributors to heart-attack risk. Women over age fifty-five have higher blood cholesterol levels than men, and women are particularly vulnerable to low levels of HDL.

Estrogen loss isn't the only contributing factor to heart disease and stroke for women as they move through perimenopause. If, as you approach menopause, you begin putting on weight, particularly around your abdomen instead of around your hips (starting to look like an "apple" instead of a "pear"), you could be significantly increasing your risk of heart disease. Other midlife diseases, such as diabetes and high blood pressure, are heavily linked to the onset of heart disease in midlife, as well.

The Dangers of Obesity and High Cholesterol

If you're courting obesity and high cholesterol, you're speeding up the effects of age on your heart's health. According to the American Heart Association's 2001 Heart and Stroke Statistical Update, nearly 34 percent of the average diet in the United States is made up of fat and over half of all Americans have high blood total cholesterol levels (over 200 mg/dl).

As women move toward menopause, their risk factors for heart disease increase dramatically, and so their vigilance and heart-healthy habits have to increase to offset the risk. Although family health history plays a role in your own likelihood of developing heart disease, you have many options for combating this deadly enemy, including diet, exercise, lifestyle changes, cholesterol-controlling medications, HRT, and more.

Heart Disease Explained

The term *heart disease* refers to any disorder or condition of the heart and blood vessels; these diseases fall under the catchall category of cardiovascular disease. Coronary artery disease is a common form of heart disease that occurs when arteries become lined with heavy deposits of plaque—a substance made up of cholesterol, calcium, and other minerals. The plaque buildup narrows the diameter of the vessels, thus limiting the amount of blood that can flow through the arteries, contributing to a condition known as atherosclerosis. Blood carries oxygen to all of the body's muscles, including the heart. As plaque narrows or blocks the coronary arteries, the heart muscle is starved of oxygen, which can damage the heart muscle itself and lead to a heart attack.

For women entering menopause, the threat of heart disease comes mainly from coronary artery disease, the atherosclerosis that contributes to it, and the heart attacks and stroke that all of these conditions can lead to.

The Symptoms of Heart Disease

Although minor symptoms can be mild or innocuous, the first major symptom you're likely to experience is a chest pain called angina—a squeezing, heaviness, or tightness in your chest that happens when your heart is starved of oxygen. As the atherosclerosis progresses, the pain of angina can become worse. Angina is your warning that you have heart disease and are at risk for suffering a heart attack.

On the other hand, unfortunately, you may have no warning at all. Many people are unaware that they suffer from any kind of heart disease until they have a heart attack, but women are more likely than men to experience the warning pangs of angina before a full heart attack occurs. Because the symptoms of angina are very much like those of a heart attack, it's critical that you report symptoms to your health-care provider immediately.

The symptoms of heart attack vary; in some cases, the attack is so minor that no noticeable symptoms occur. In fact, many heart attacks in women are misdiagnosed as heartburn, indigestion, or gall bladder problems. But in many other cases, the symptoms of heart attack are evident, including a crushing or dull pain in the chest; pain in the left shoulder, arm, neck, or back; sweating, nausea, shortness of breath; fatigue or dizziness; or burning pain in the mid-chest.

When a Heart Attack Hits

If one or more of your coronary arteries become completely blocked, you can have a heart attack. Over 200,000 women die of heart attack every year in this country, and many thousand more suffer an attack and survive. A heart attack can be mild, moderate, or severe, depending upon the amount of damage to the heart muscle. If only a small area of the heart is deprived of blood, the healthy heart tissue surrounding it continues to work, allowing the damaged part of the heart to heal as new vessels grow in from the healthy areas. But if damage occurs in several of these small areas, they can combine to damage the heart beyond repair.

Only rarely do heart attacks cause the heart to stop functioning completely. More often, you have a chance to make a big difference in the amount of damage your heart receives and your chances for a recovery. But you must act quickly; most heart attack damage occurs within the first two hours after you feel the pain. If you have any reason to suspect you may be having an attack—a personal history of angina or a family history of heart disease—be prepared to get help. If there was ever a situation where the old "better safe than sorry" expression applies, this is it. Be smart. Get medical attention immediately.

Plaque Buildup Contributes to Strokes

Atherosclerosis can also contribute to the plaque buildup in the carotid arteries that carry oxygen-rich blood to the brain. The plaque buildup can lead to the formation of blood clots, which can break loose from the inside of the vessel walls and be carried to your brain, causing a stroke. In 1998, stroke killed twice as many American women as were killed by breast cancer.

Women, Menopause, and Heart Disease

One in five women has some type of heart or blood vessel disease. Women in their childbearing years are statistically less prone to heart disease than are men of the same age. According to the American Heart Association, "Menopause itself appears to increase a woman's risks of coronary heart disease and stroke." If your menopause occurs naturally, the risk rises slowly. But if menopause results from surgery, the risks can rise dramatically and quickly.

To understand why women's postmenopausal risk of heart disease surpasses that of men, it's important to understand some of the root causes of heart disease. One of the most important contributors to heart disease is high blood cholesterol levels. When you develop high blood cholesterol levels, you have too much artery-clogging fat in your bloodstream. The diminished supply of estrogen that occurs with menopause, weight gain, and the aging of your cardiovascular system all contribute to developing high cholesterol levels.

Do ERT and HRT Lower Your Risk?

A number of medical researchers and scientists believe that a woman's own natural estrogen might help protect her from heart disease, but they're still studying how the hormone may have that effect. Estrogen plays an important role in maintaining healthy, strong muscle tissue, including the muscle of the heart. Estrogen also has an impact on the blood's level of triglycerides and low-density lipoproteins (LDL) or "bad" cholesterol, both of which can contribute to atherosclerosis and heart attack. Some studies have shown that estrogen contributes to healthy, reactive arteries and an increased blood flow. As a result, blood vessels are better able to relax and respond to exercise and physical stress by dilating and providing more blood flow when needed.

According to the American Heart Association (AHA), estrogen replacement therapy (ERT) does have a positive effect on several risk factors for heart disease and stroke. For example, oral forms of both ERT and HRT increase the level of HDL cholesterol and lower the level of LDL cholesterol. Estrogen administered in the form of a skin patch also has some beneficial effects on your lipid profile, although it may take longer for these benefits to show up on your blood tests. Even so, the AHA doesn't recommend that you use either of these therapies as a replacement for cholesterol-lowering drugs if you're battling high blood cholesterol levels.

One twenty-five-year-long study, known as the Harvard Nurses' Health Study, linked ERT and HRT with a lower risk of death from heart disease—a benefit that lasted even after ten years of hormone treatment. Another study, the Heart and Estrogen-Progestin Replacement Study (HERS), focused on postmenopausal women who already had coronary heart disease. After approximately four years of follow-up, that study indicated that HRT did not reduce the participants' overall risk of heart attack or death from coronary heart disease as much as previously expected, nor did it have any major impact on their overall risk of stroke. Results of a new, ongoing study funded by the NIH actually found a small but increased risk of nonfatal heart attack, stroke, deep vein blood clot, and pulmonary embolus in women taking one form of HRT for several years. An increased risk of stroke has also been shown in women taking estrogen alone.

Studies continue and you can expect new developments in our understanding of the role of estrogen, estrogen replacement, and heart disease in women. For now, you need to weigh your own individual potential benefits and risks of any treatment for heart disease, and discuss them carefully with your health-care provider.

The Risk Factors You Own

There are few key risk factors for developing heart disease that cannot be controlled. However, women face two unchangeable risks:

- **Growing older:** The older you get, the greater your risk for developing heart disease. Four out of five people who die of it are sixty-five or older. And the older women are when they suffer a heart attack, the more likely they are to die of it.
- **Heredity:** If your parents had heart disease, you're more likely to develop it. Sometimes it is because of a propensity to high cholesterol levels. Race-associated conditions can have an impact on heart disease risk, as well. Because African Americans can have

more severe high blood pressure, they have an elevated risk for developing coronary heart disease. Mexican Americans, Native Americans, Asian Americans, and native Hawaiians also have higher risk.

Having these unchangeable risk factors doesn't mean you're destined to suffer from heart disease. But it does mean that you need to be extra vigilant about controlling the risks you can change.

High Cholesterol

High blood cholesterol is a major risk factor for developing heart disease. After menopause, women tend to develop high levels of triglycerides (a form of fat), in addition to high levels of low-density lipoprotein (LDL) cholesterol. At the same time, their levels of high-density lipoprotein (HDL) can diminish. All of these factors lead to out-of-balance blood cholesterol levels, too much fat in the bloodstream, and the buildup of artery-clogging plaque in the pathways that channel oxygen-rich blood to the heart and brain. For every 1 percent reduction in elevated blood cholesterol levels, you get a 2 to 3 percent reduction in your chances of having a heart attack.

Cholesterol is a natural, essential substance in the bloodstream. The fraction of your total cholesterol that is HDL cholesterol is a protein that helps keep all fats and cholesterols moving through your bloodstream (and not glued to your arterial walls), so it actually helps you stave off a potential heart attack. LDL cholesterol moves cholesterol through the rest of your body—but it also has a tendency to linger in your arteries and stick to the walls. Elevated levels of triglycerides may or may not indicate that you're headed for a heart attack, but their levels also need to be monitored.

Your total blood cholesterol level should remain below 200 mg/dl (milligrams per deciliter of blood); anything over 239 mg/dl needs to be considered a high risk. Here's how the individual cholesterol numbers should stack up:

- **HDL:** More than 60 mg/dl is good; less than 35 mg/dl puts you at high risk.
- **LDL:** Less than 130 mg/dl is desirable, up to 159 mg/dl is considered borderline high, and 160 mg/dl and higher is high risk.
- **Triglycerides:** Less than 200 mg/dl is considered normal, up to 400 mg/dl is borderline high, 400 to 1,000 mg/dl is high, and over 1,000 mg/dl is way too high.

A low-fat diet and regular exercise can help most people maintain healthy blood cholesterol levels. Where those efforts fall short, studies have shown that a variety of cholesterol-lowering drugs, called statins, do actually reduce your risk of dying from a heart disease. Although some of these drugs may have side effects, the medications currently on the market are considered safe and effective. Consult your physician; do not rely on a homeopath or other alternative health care if your lipid profile is abnormal.

The effectiveness of HRT and ERT in managing blood cholesterol is still the subject of much medical research. Estrogen has been shown to reduce total blood cholesterol levels and to raise levels of HDL. But recent studies indicate that some types of estrogen may slightly increase levels of triglycerides in the bloodstream. Your triglycerides may decrease if the estrogen in your prescription regimen is combined with just the right progestin for HRT. Though the AHA doesn't recommend ERT or HRT as a first defense against high cholesterol, you should discuss this option with your health-care provider, who can make recommendations based on your complete health profile, family medical history, and current symptoms.

High Blood Pressure

High blood pressure (hypertension) is another silent plague of women age fifty-five and over. More than half of all women in that age group have blood pressure greater than 140/90 (the high-blood-pressure threshold), but few feel its effects. In fact, though some estimates say that one in four people in the United States suffers from high blood pressure, nearly one-third of those individuals are unaware of their condition. Even if you have had normal blood pressure all of your life, you might develop high blood pressure after menopause. Having high blood pressure makes you a prime candidate for developing heart disease. It also contributes to kidney disease and can lead to congestive heart failure, heart attack, and stroke.

Blood pressure results from the force of your heart pumping your blood through your veins. If you exercise or become excited, your heart rate increases, sending more blood through your system. If your arteries are clean and wide open, the blood flows freely; if they're narrow or blocked, the buildup of blood trying to course through your veins puts pressure on the arterial walls—that's high blood pressure. If your arteries are clean and healthy, your blood pressure rises for a short period of time, then returns to normal as the blood moves through your circulatory system. If you have hypertension, however, your blood pressure is greater than 140/90, even when you're at rest; the extra pressure on your heart and arteries never lets up. If high blood pressure occurs in a person with atherosclerosis, the walls of the vessels are toughened and less elastic, and even less able to cope with stress.

Encouraging Declines in Cardiovascular Disease

Between 1988 and 1998, death rates from coronary heart disease in women declined by approximately 25 percent, and death rates from all cardiovascular diseases in women declined by nearly 19 percent. These drops are probably due to increased awareness of heart disease incidence in women and earlier diagnosis through cholesterol screening.

Most doctors consider between 120/80 and 130/90 the ideal blood pressure reading. Though some people have suffered from low blood pressure, it's a relatively uncommon occurrence and not life threatening. Regular exercise and a diet high in vegetables and fruit, but low in sodium, can help control high blood pressure. If diet, exercise, and weight loss (when indicated) don't bring blood pressure down, your health-care provider may prescribe drug therapy.

Medications for Blood Pressure and Cholesterol Management

Though diet and exercise are your two most effective means for controlling cholesterol levels and blood pressure, many medications are currently available to treat both conditions:

- **Simvastatin, Pravastatin, and Lovastatin** are just some of the cholesterol-controlling drugs that fall within a category known as HMG-CoA reductase inhibitors. These drugs work by blocking an enzyme that your body uses to produce cholesterol, and they have been shown to be effective in lowering cholesterol levels and preventing deaths due to heart disease. These drugs can interact with some other medications, and they aren't often recommended for people with active liver disease. If you are hesitant about beginning statin therapy, get a copy of your blood test result and consult another physician for a second opinion.

- **Diuretics** (including thiazides, potassium-sparing diuretics, and loop diuretics) flush water and sodium from the body and can be effective for reducing blood pressure. Diuretics reduce the level of fluid in your bloodstream and help remove sodium from your circulation, so they may help open up arteries and boost the capacity of your arterial system and thereby lower blood pressure against your arterial walls. Their effect is temporary and limited, and they don't have any long-term benefit on your arteries' or kidneys' health. If you do not have high blood pressure and don't have a tendency to retain water, they may not be appropriate for you.

- **Beta blockers**, including lopranonol and metroprolol, block some of the nerve impulses to the heart; as a result, the heartbeat slows and the heart's workload decreases. Doctors often prescribe beta blockers along with diuretics to control blood pressure. Sometimes beta blockers are combined with alpha blockers—drugs that relax blood vessels—in one medication called an alpha-beta blocker. Labetalol is one example of these alpha-beta blocking drugs. All of these medications are extremely powerful, and therefore are carefully prescribed and monitored by doctors and other medical professionals. Make sure to tell your doctor if you are following or not following a low-sodium diet, when prescribed.

- **ACE inhibitors** are also effective in controlling high blood pressure, and they seem to work by inhibiting the formation of the hormone angiotensin II—a substance that causes blood vessels to constrict. Researchers are still trying to determine exactly how these drugs work to lower blood pressure, but some doctors are prescribing them for that purpose.

High blood pressure medications have a range of possible side effects, and most doctors recommend other methods as a first line of defense against this disease. Combination (multi-drug) therapy is common nowadays, but following the advice of one primary-care physician is best.

Diabetes

Diabetes is another heart disease risk factor that is of particular concern to women. Nearly 6 million women in the United States have been diagnosed with diabetes, and another 2.5 million women have undiagnosed diabetes. Having diabetes ups your risk of heart disease and stroke by two to four times. Every year, over 60,000 Americans die of complications of diabetes, and the disease can lead to a host of other conditions, including kidney failure, blindness, and nerve disease.

Diabetes mellitus occurs when the body is unable to produce adequate amounts of insulin or efficiently use the insulin it produces (insulin resistance). Insulin is produced in the pancreas, and the body uses it to process the sugar and carbohydrates you consume into energy. Type 2 or adult onset diabetes is the most common form of the disease, and it usually occurs at middle age.

Researchers don't know what causes the development of diabetes, and no drug can cure it. However, diabetes can be controlled—and sometimes disappears altogether—through diet, exercise, and weight loss. Statistics show that 80 to 90 percent of people with diabetes are overweight, and many have high blood pressure and/or lead inactive lives. Though a large number of diabetics require insulin or drug therapy, many others are able to control their disease through behavior modification, such as diet, exercise, and weight loss.

Obesity

The numbers of obese people in the United States continue to rise at alarming levels. The percentage of overweight Americans has risen by over 60 percent in the past decade, and nearly half of all American women are overweight or obese—conditions defined in general by a body weight more than 30 percent over the ideal for the body's height and frame, or having an abnormally high body mass index (BMI; see Chapter 13 for chart).

Though obesity can result in obvious emotional distress, its health-damaging effects are even more insidious. Although still under study, some research indicates that nearly 70 percent of diagnosed cases of heart disease may be directly linked to obesity. And obesity is a gateway disease for numerous other conditions, including diabetes, high blood pressure, high blood cholesterol levels, kidney disease, sleep apnea, depression, menstrual irregularities, joint disease, and even some forms of cancer.

The Effects of Smoking on Your Heart

Smoking tobacco is hard on your entire body, but it delivers a particularly hard blow to your heart. Each time you draw in a lungful of tobacco smoke, you temporarily increase your heart rate and blood pressure and deplete the oxygen in your bloodstream that should be going to feed your heart and other body tissues. If you're a smoker, the best thing you can do for your heart—and the rest of your body—is to stop smoking now.

Though weight gain in middle age isn't uncommon for both men and women, women are at special risk for heart disease from their postmenopausal weight gain. As previously noted, many women tend to add weight in their abdomen and upper body during menopause.

This type of fat seems to be linked closely with a number of other risk factors for heart disease, including diabetes.

Our sex, age, individual biological and genetic makeup, psychological condition, and environment each appear capable of playing a major role in the development of obesity. Still, behavior modification is a powerful weapon against obesity. A low-calorie, low-fat, high-fiber diet and regular exercise are the first defenses against this disease. But for many people, other methods prove helpful, including drug therapy, psychotherapy, hypnosis, acupuncture, and even surgery. As this disease continues to become more prevalent in our society, look for further discoveries and advancement in its treatment.

Controlling Your Risks

Though you might have a genetic susceptibility to high blood pressure, high cholesterol, or diabetes, or your age may increase your chances of contracting heart disease, you can take positive action to manage your overall risks. Here are some suggestions:

- **Eat a low-fat, low-cholesterol, high-fiber diet.** The less saturated fat you consume, the better you'll be able to manage blood cholesterol levels. Try to build your diet around fresh fruits, vegetables, and whole grains. Limit the amount of fat, meat, and dairy products you consume, and go easy on the salt—especially if you suffer from high blood pressure. And eat some soy; eating 25 grams of soy protein—from soy milk, veggie burgers, or tofu—a day can help lower your LDL cholesterol level by as much as 5 to 10 percent.
- **Manage your weight.** Ask your health-care provider to help you determine what your weight should be and how you can best reach and maintain that weight. The first step to weight

management is diet management. No matter what other lifestyle changes you make, being overweight or obese can dramatically increase your risks of suffering from some form of heart disease.

- **Exercise regularly.** Physical activity not only helps control obesity, it also helps dramatically reduce the severity of many conditions that contribute to heart disease. The Surgeon General recommends thirty minutes of exercise, at least three days a week, but an hour of exercise, four days a week is better. Your exercise should boost your heart rate, but it doesn't have to be a "killer" routine. Try to combine both weight training (such as lifting weights) and aerobic (swimming, walking, running) exercises, preceded and followed by a series of stretching movements.

- **Drink alcohol in moderation.** Keep your consumption to no more than one drink a day.

- **Stop smoking.** Now—use whatever means necessary.

Keep Smokers Outside

In 1999, the *New England Journal of Medicine* reported a study that found that nonsmokers exposed to environmental smoke have a higher risk of coronary heart disease than those who aren't. So don't be shy—ask smokers to smoke outside.

- **Find ways to avoid or relieve stress.** When you're under stress, your heart rate can go up, your breathing can become shallow, and all of your muscles can become tense. If you want your heart and brain to be nourished by a strong, healthy flow of oxygenated blood, learn to keep stress to a minimum. Exercise helps, as does relaxation therapy, meditation, and quiet time spent enjoying the things you love.

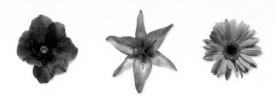

chapter nine | **What You Should Know about Osteoporosis**

Osteoporosis—the loss of bone mass that results in porous, fragile bones—threatens nearly 28 million people in the United States, 80 percent of whom are women. According to the National Osteoporosis Foundation, 8 million women have osteoporosis and millions more have low bone density. Half of all women over the age of fifty will suffer an osteoporosis-related bone fracture at some time during their lives. Most of these fractures are preventable if a doctor diagnoses the early stages of osteoporosis, called osteopenia, at a time when preventable measures are possible.

Estrogen helps prevent the loss of bone density, and that's what makes osteoporosis such a growing threat for menopausal women. Hip and wrist fractures, collapsing vertebrae (the small bones that make up your spine), and the familiar stooped posture of many elderly women are just some of the all-too-common effects of this disease. Any bone in the body can crumble when this disease progresses to an advanced state.

A fractured hip or collapsed vertebrae caused by mild trauma might be the first outright symptom of osteoporosis. Unfortunately, by the time such a break occurs, the disease has already done damage to your body's framework. Health-care providers, therefore, depend on family medical history and sound prevention methods to stop osteoporosis before it strikes. Beyond age, low estrogen levels, and family history, risk factors include a small, thin frame; a diet low in calcium; or a history of eating disorders such as anorexia or bulimia (in which estrogen levels usually drop and menstrual periods often cease); and taking certain medications, including steroids (such as prednisone), anticonvulsants, thyroid hormone replacement therapy, or lithium, for more than three months.

African-American women have a much lower incidence of post-menopausal osteoporosis than do Northern European and Asian women. However, they still need the same screening for other risk factors.

Osteoporosis Explained

When you're a child, your bones have a lot of growing to do, so your body produces much more new bone than it takes back in through resorption (the process of absorbing old bone cells back into the body).

Around age thirty, your body reaches a stage of peak bone mass, where your bones are as large and dense as they will ever be. At that stage, resorption slowly begins to outpace bone production. If resorption becomes too rapid or if bone cell production becomes too slow, you're at risk for developing osteoporosis. If you didn't build your bones to their optimum size during the years leading to peak bone mass, your risk is even greater.

The loss of bone calcium speeds up dramatically as estrogen levels drop off during perimenopause. By the time you've reached perimenopause, you've passed the age when you could continue to develop a stronger, healthier skeleton. Your goals should then be to slow calcium loss and maintain your bones' current strength.

Currently, there is no cure for osteoporosis. But you can slow the progress of the disease dramatically through a treatment plan involving some combination of medication, diet, and exercise. Recent experiments with drugs that may actually help rebuild lost bone tissue offer true encouragement to victims of this disease and those who treat them. But remember, prevention is easier than treatment.

How Osteoporosis Strikes

Bone tissue loss isn't painful in its early stages—everyone experiences it every day. Weak bones don't ache, or creak, or exhibit any other kind of warning. In fact, even after someone suffers a bone fracture, if she and her doctor don't suspect osteoporosis and follow up with the proper diagnostic tests, the disease can remain undiagnosed and untreated.

Osteoporotic bones lose mass very slowly; over time, the bones become so fragile that they can break under very slight strain. If the broken bone goes unnoticed or the break is apparent but no one connects it to the disease, osteoporosis continues to erode the bones until another fracture occurs. By the time the warning flag goes up, the disease may have advanced to a critical stage.

Diagnosing the Disease

A close review of your osteoporosis risk profile will tell your health-care provider how soon (and often) you need to be checked for the development of the disease. The most common and effective diagnostic tool for osteoporosis is a bone density measurement known as a bone mineral density (BMD) test. BMD tests can measure the density of the bones in your spine, wrist, heel, and/or hip.

The Risks of Osteoporosis-Related Fractures

Osteoporosis-related fractures can be killers. In 1991, nearly 300,000 Americans age forty-five and older were hospitalized as a result of hip fractures, and osteoporosis was a contributor to most of these breaks. On average, 24 percent of patients who experience a hip fracture after the age of fifty die within the year that follows their fracture.

A dual energy X-ray absorptiometry (DEXA) test is typically used to measure bone density. In this test, low-dose X-ray beams scan your lower (lumbar) spine and/or hips for ten to twenty minutes. The test isn't painful, and you're exposed to minimal radiation, so it's safe and effective. Other types of bone density scans use ultrasound to measure the bone mass in your heel or wrist, but aren't as conclusive as the DEXA test. However, a quick office scan of the density of your heel or wrist still provides useful knowledge, especially if you are relatively young (less than forty-five years old) and have risk factors for this condition.

Besides warning you about osteoporosis before you suffer a fracture, bone density tests can help you determine your rate of bone loss and help you gauge the effectiveness of your efforts to slow that loss. A BMD test can tell you how your bone density compares to that of healthy bone tissue from a person of your age and—more importantly—to that of an average twenty-five-year-old.

Menopause and Osteoporosis

As you approach menopause, your chances for developing osteoporosis increase dramatically. Your bones are in a constant state of remodeling its bone tissue, by removing old bone tissue cells through resorption and creating new ones. But, as with many remodelers, the body is more adept at tearing down the old than at building the new. Your body depends upon its growth hormones—especially estrogen—to help pace the remodeling process.

Exercising as Prevention

Exercise not only helps maintain your bones' health but also keeps your joints and muscles flexible and strong. Those improvements go a long way toward helping you prevent fractures caused by falls. But exercise alone won't prevent osteoporosis. If you combine a sensible exercise program with a well-balanced diet and avoid smoking and excess alcohol consumption, you'll go a long way to preserving your bone health, even after menopause.

Estrogen Loss Depletes Bone Tissue

Estrogen protects your bones by controlling the amount of bone removed by resorption. When your estrogen levels drop after menopause (either gradually through natural menopause or dramatically as a result of induced menopause), your bones lose that protection. As a result, in the five to eight years following menopause, your bone loss can increase dramatically as your body adjusts to the loss of ovarian estrogen.

If you've gone through an early menopause, your body has endured a greater-than-normal estrogen loss and your risk of experiencing accelerated bone loss increases. And if you've ever experienced extensive or frequent bouts of amenorrhea (lack of periods), your bones have been through periods of accelerated bone loss due to a loss of estrogen protection.

The Facts about Postmenopausal Bone Loss

The average woman loses up to 3 percent of bone mass a year after menopause. According to the National Osteoporosis Foundation, women can lose up to 20 percent of their bone mass in just the first five to seven years following menopause.

So does that mean that every woman emerges from the first decade of menopause with thin, fragile bones? Certainly not! Remember that the condition of your bones plays a role in preserving their mass, as do a number of other factors, including heredity, environment, diet, and exercise.

When Hyperparathyroidism Contributes to Osteoporosis

Your parathyroid gland secretes a hormone that controls the amount of calcium released by your bones into the bloodstream. Rarely, this gland becomes overactive (hyperparathyroidism), and your bones can release too much calcium and contribute to the development of osteoporosis. This condition is particularly dangerous for women in menopause. The good news is that hyperparathyroidism is a treatable condition.

Every woman—regardless of her age or health—needs to understand her risks for developing osteoporosis and have a sound, ongoing plan for maintaining bone health. Waiting until you're older or waiting until you've entered menopause to protect yourself against osteoporosis won't work; by then, you could already be losing the battle against bone loss.

Eating for Strong Bones

Your body stores pounds of calcium in its bones, and calcium is an essential nutrient for all of your body's organs and tissues. Eating a well-balanced diet with adequate amounts of calcium and vitamin D won't guarantee an osteoporosis-free life, but it's the best method for helping your body prevent or slow the disease. For more information on the importance of calcium, also see Chapter 13.

Lifestyle choices such as excess consumption of alcohol and caffeine, inadequate calcium and vitamin D intake, cigarette smoking, and a lack of weight-bearing exercise can all contribute to the development of osteoporosis over time. Take steps to control these risks, and if you're at high risk for osteoporosis, get regular bone density tests. Older women should also have their height checked: Although perhaps you were 5'6" in high school, you might be surprised at what you measure out to be now in the doctor's office. Your doctor might not automatically offer this, so ask if need be.

Using Estrogen for Bone Health

Most doctors agree that estrogen therapy can halt bone loss after menopause and may actually contribute to bone growth. Estrogen helps to activate the vitamin D in your body to enhance its ability to absorb calcium. It also promotes the production of collagen in your system that aids in the development of bone strength and flexibility.

Bone Health for Vegetarians

If you're a vegetarian, you must eat a well-balanced diet of beans, seeds, grains, and a broad variety of vegetables for a bone-healthy diet. Ovo-lacto vegetarians eat eggs and dairy products and therefore have more access to calcium in their diet. If you eat no dairy products at all, you need to carefully monitor your calcium intake and consider supplements.

Estrogen replacement therapy (ERT) has been shown to reduce bone loss, increase bone density in the spine and hip, and reduce the risk of hip fractures in postmenopausal women. If you are approaching menopause, talk to your health-care professional about the benefits and risks of estrogen for the prevention of osteoporosis after menopause. ERT is also beneficial for the heart, eyes, brain, colon, and joints, so try to touch on all these areas with your physician.

Alternatives for Managing Bone Loss

Though estrogen is the undisputed queen of bone maintenance, medical science has made a number of strides in finding alternative drugs for slowing the bone deterioration associated with the estrogen deficiency of menopause. The following medications are other options for preventing or slowing the progress of osteoporosis:

- **Alendronate:** an FDA-approved biphosphonate that helps slow the breakdown of bone tissue that occurs in osteoporosis. According to the American College of Obstetrics and Gynecology, research trials on this drug have shown that it not only helps slow bone loss but also may even build bone tissue in the spine and hip—two areas most prone to the complications of osteoporosis and possible fracture. Alendronate has been associated with irritation of the esophagus in a small percentage of patients, but new dosages and formulations are under development that will reduce its potential for negative side effects. A new once-a-week dosage significantly reduces short-term side effects and makes the patient precautions easier to follow.
- **Risedronate:** a drug that inhibits the body's ability to reabsorb bone tissue, and thereby slows bone loss. Risedronate doesn't seem to cause as much stomach or esophageal irritation as alendronate. It also protects the bone density of the total body and reduces the risk of fracture in the spinal vertebrae and the hip, especially in high-risk women.

- **Calcitonin:** not really a nonhormonal treatment for osteoporosis but a hormone produced by the parathyroid gland, calcitonin is available as a prescription drug. Calcitonin helps slow bone loss by slowing bone resorption in a process similar to the previous two drugs in this list. Typically, calcitonin is given as a nasal spray that you take two times a day, which does decrease the risk of side effects, especially to the esophagus. It has been shown to be useful in reducing the risk of fractures of the spinal vertebrae in very elderly women; it does not lessen the risk of hip fracture or protect younger women.

- **Raloxifene:** although it doesn't quite fit as a "nonhormonal" approach to fighting osteoporosis—an artificial hormone used as an alternative to estrogen. Raloxifene was approved by the FDA for the prevention of osteoporosis, and studies have shown that it maintains bone density in some women (though not quite as well as estrogen) and may prevent fractures of the spine but not the hip. Raloxifene may cause hot flashes, and though it lowers LDL cholesterol, it doesn't raise HDL cholesterol. It is not considered as beneficial as estrogen for the bone or the heart.

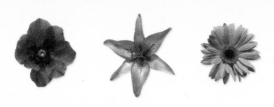

chapter ten | $\mathscr{P}$erimenopause and Moods

Your emotional health and physical health are closely linked. This connection is never more keenly felt than during menopause and the years immediately preceding and following it. Many women experience a series of physical, chemical, and social changes during perimenopause that can shake their self-confidence and threaten their emotional health. But you have a remarkable ability to control the speed and severity of those changes.

Looking Stress in the Eye

During midlife, women face any number of stressors, including career and financial issues, body image changes, emerging health problems, divorce, widowhood, struggles with teenage children, and increasing responsibilities for aging parents. Though many women will have dealt with these issues at previous times in life, the added stress of adjusting to hormonal fluctuations, hot flashes, weight gain, or other potential side effects of perimenopause can make the burden of stress harder to bear during midlife.

Stress can contribute to and exacerbate a range of medical and emotional problems, from stomach disorders, headaches, forgetfulness, and insomnia, to mood swings, anxiety, and even depression. Unless you find ways to eliminate or manage stress, you won't be successful in combating the mood-related problems you may experience during perimenopause. If you suffer from these difficulties, your first step toward recovery is identifying the sources of stress in your life.

Managing Stress

You can't avoid all sources of stress, but you may be able to work around many of them. For example, if a hectic work and family schedule is depleting your energy and contributing to stress, see what activities you can trim from your daily list, and ask your partner and children for help. Learn to delegate whatever "to do" items those around you can handle, rather than suffer in silence. And don't stop at examining your home and family responsibilities, either. Evaluate your job and work habits to spot stress fixes there, as well. Ask your boss for more flexible work times, find someone to carpool with, or even arrange to work at home one day a week.

Stay in Touch with Your Emotions

As you move into perimenopause, it's important that you remain aware of your feelings and alert for signs of emotional problems. Just as you have to check up on and monitor your physical health regularly, you need to watch for and deal with symptoms of emotional disorder to maintain your overall fitness and well-being.

When you've pinpointed and reduced the stressors that you can control, find ways to cope with the stress you can't get rid of. Exercise regularly, spend time engaged in leisure activities you enjoy, eat a healthy diet, and go easy on your mind and body—don't expect to perform every task flawlessly and on time.

Stress presents a real health risk you simply cannot overlook. It will wear you out, age your body and mind, drain your spirit, and cause serious and lasting health problems. Talk to your doctor, a therapist, a counselor, a friend, a minister, or a trusted family member, and ask for help in finding ways to manage stress.

The Menopause-Mood Connection

Many researchers believe that the fluctuating levels of estrogen and progesterone many women experience during perimenopause can contribute to mood swings and other emotional symptoms. Though the mechanisms of their impact are under continual study, doctors do know that estrogen is directly related to our body's production of serotonin—an important chemical that works in the brain to regulate moods. As estrogen levels shift, so does the brain's supply of serotonin—therefore, moods can shift, as well. Keep a journal and see if your mood swings are related to your menstrual cycle, even if your periods are occurring irregularly. If a pattern emerges, your doctor can help you address it, and not necessarily with medication.

Body chemistry isn't the only thing that can trigger midlife mood decay. Women who are dealing with changing roles at home or at work, changing levels of energy, or diminishing feelings of general fitness and well-being are at risk of suffering from emotional upheavals and imbalances.

Stay Optimistic

Though no conclusive studies have proven the benefits of optimism, many medical professionals have observed pessimistic patients are prone to have an elevated blood pressure, less resistance to disease, and a slower recovery time following illnesses or injury.

Coming to grips with your emotional upsets by recognizing symptoms and tracking them to their source can be a first step toward resolving the problem. You may be able to control mild mood disturbances simply by changing your diet, exercise program, or reactions to certain stress-inducing stimuli. Such techniques are covered later in this chapter along with information about medication, counseling, and other treatment options that can help restore your emotional order and balance when lifestyle and behavioral changes aren't enough.

Tracking Your Mood Swings

Mood shifts are relatively mild changes that can quickly take a woman from feelings of joy to anger, fatigue, or despair. The emotional triggers for these responses can be unpredictable—and, sometimes, seemingly inconsequential. Perimenopausal women who report mood swings cite a wide range of stimuli for these events, whether it be bursting into tears when a certain song comes on the radio or becoming incredibly angry when children or a partner fails to take care of their household responsibilities. Mood swings can sometimes be no more than a natural response, magnified to a level much higher than normal.

Mood swings can also be a response to a medical condition or chemical imbalance in your body that can, perhaps, be treated through counseling, medication, or other therapy. Although you can expect to experience some mood swings in your life, frequent or severe mood swings can create problems with family, coworkers, and friends; cause missed workdays; discourage participation in social functions or enjoyable activities; or create feelings of alienation, exhaustion, fear, and a lack of control. If mood swings are so severe that they get in the way of your full—and fulfilling—life, take action to control them.

The Symptoms of Anxiety

Anxiety is a natural, healthy response to certain realities of life—beginning a new job, meeting deadlines, passing examinations, and so on. But anxiety that interferes with your ability to function at full capacity throughout your day and then sleep soundly throughout the night is definitely unhealthy.

Panic Attacks

Women in perimenopause sometimes report the occurrence of panic attacks—overwhelming feelings of intense fear or impending doom that occur suddenly and repeatedly, for no good reason. Symptoms include shortness of breath, choking sensations, heart pounding or palpitations, and the sensation of losing control.

Anxiety can be associated with depression, or it can be a side effect of sleeplessness, excess fatigue, or unmanageable levels of stress. Many people suffering from anxiety describe it as overwhelming feelings of fear, nervousness, or the conviction that something dreadful is about to happen—though they often can't pinpoint what that something may be. When these feelings go unchecked and begin to interfere with normal, everyday functioning, they may indicate an anxiety disorder. Some other symptoms of anxiety include:

- Chest pain, racing heartbeat, or fast breathing
- Stomach pain, cramps, or diarrhea
- Hand-wringing, pacing, or other repetitive nervous movement

Anxiety disorders include social phobias, such as agoraphobia (fear of going out in public), specific phobias (such as fear of dogs or spiders), or obsessive behaviors (such as obsessive hand washing or repeatedly checking door locks or appliance switches).

Menopause and Depression

Are you certain to suffer from depression as you approach menopause? Absolutely not. However, women who have a family or personal history of depression are more at risk for suffering from depression during perimenopause. The connection between this period of transition and depression can be both physical and emotional. In order to understand that connection better, you first need to understand exactly what depression is—and how it differs from mood swings and minor bouts of "the blues."

What Is Depression?

There's a world of difference between passing feelings of disappointment, dissatisfaction, or sadness and an ongoing state of major depression. According to the *Journal of the American Medical Association*, between 5 and 10 percent of the U.S. population experiences major depression; nearly 25 percent of all women will suffer from depression at some point during their lives.

Many women in perimenopause have minor mood problems that may include insomnia, anxiety, and irritability. But when these problems become severe or long-standing, these women can develop major depression.

Mood Swings Pass

Women approaching menopause often (but not always) report anxiety and panic attacks, bouts of sadness, or unexplained surges of elation. These emotional swings tend to be erratic and transient, not long-lived facts of life for perimenopausal women.

Another, less severe, type of depression is known as dysthymia. The symptoms of dysthymia are similar to those of major depression and may be chronic and long-term, but they aren't disabling. Finally, people suffering from bipolar disorder (manic-depressive illness) experience extreme mood shifts that swing wildly between manic highs and depressed lows.

Know the Symptoms

Though transient feelings of sadness, despair, or general dissatisfaction with life are common during perimenopause, if these feelings are long-lasting or severe, they could signal depression.

Depression makes itself known to each individual in unique ways, but some symptoms are typical. The National Institute of Mental Health provides a list of common symptoms of depression (though few people suffer all of them). Here are some of those symptoms:

- Feeling persistently sad, anxious, empty, hopeless, or pessimistic.
- Experiencing a strong sense of impending doom, with no idea what form this awful event might take or why it will happen.
- Losing interest in hobbies or activities you once enjoyed (including sex).
- Feeling guilty, worthless, or helpless.
- Losing energy and feeling fatigued and slowed down.
- Suffering from insomnia, early morning awakening, or oversleeping.
- Experiencing a dramatic change in appetite or weight.
- Difficulty concentrating, remembering, or making decisions.
- Having thoughts of suicide and death or suicide attempts.
- Suffering from persistent physical symptoms (headache, pain, digestive disorders) that don't respond to treatment.

If you suffer from depression, the sooner you get help, the more quickly and effectively you can overcome the physical and emotional side effects of this devastating condition. Your goal is to get your life back in balance so you can regain your sense of confidence and purpose.

Pinpoint the Causes of Depression

No one cause is at the source of every case of depression, but it usually is associated with a change in the brain's structure or functions. Sometimes a vulnerability to depression is genetically inherited, but depression can be brought on by physical changes from stress, injury, illness, an accident, or a severe emotional event. Some people have genuine cause to be depressed, such as a reaction to a divorce or death of a loved one. Healing from severe trauma takes time. Hormonal shifts, such as those women experience in pregnancy, perimenopause, and menopause, can also contribute to depression in women.

Recognize Your Risks

If you have a predisposition to this illness, don't ignore feelings of depression that arise as you near the age of menopause. Talk to your doctor, therapist, or other health-care professional about your concerns; it's much easier to treat earlier than later.

Menopause doesn't cause depression, but the hormonal changes of perimenopause can join with other natural life events of middle age to contribute to a depressed state. Women who have suffered in the past from depression or who have experienced severe PMS seem to be especially vulnerable to depression during perimenopause.

Medical problems, such as thyroid disorders, as well as the use of some medications, such as those used to treat hypertension, can trigger mood swings, depression, and anxiety or make these conditions worse. Your doctor or health-care provider can review your medications and health history and uncover contributing medical conditions, such as insomnia, sleep apnea, or extreme hormonal imbalances, which may contribute to your mood swings.

Explore Your Treatment Options

Treatment options are determined, in part, by the severity of your problem and your personal and family medical history. If you suffer from major depression, your doctor is likely to prescribe some sort of antidepressant medication. Following is a quick list of some of the most commonly prescribed antidepressant and antianxiety medications:

- **Selective serotonin reuptake inhibitors (SSRIs)**, including fluoxetine, sertraline, and paroxetine (marketed as Prozac, Zoloft, and Paxil). Though SSRIs can cause depressed sexual response and other side effects in certain individuals, they are nonaddictive and work by helping your body make better use of the serotonin it naturally produces. They are designed to be taken long-term, usually for weeks or months at a time. Fluoxetine is also approved for premenstrual dysphoric disorder (PMDD, see Chapter 1) and is available as a once-a-week timed-release dosage.
- **Antianxiety drugs, or anxiolytics**—such as lorazepam (Ativan) and alprazolam (Xanax)—can lessen the effects of panic attacks, acute anxiety, and sleeplessness, and they also can treat the symptoms of PMDD that many perimenopausal women experience. Anxiolytics can have a slightly sedative effect, so many doctors prescribe them only for short periods of time. Generally these drugs are taken on an as-needed basis.

Psychological counseling—psychotherapy—is a powerful treatment option for women experiencing excess anxiety, stress, or mood disturbance during perimenopause and menopause. Most studies have shown that counseling in conjunction with antidepressant medication offers more long-term and effective results than does a treatment using medication alone. Interpersonal therapy and cognitive-behavioral therapy are most commonly used to treat emotional problems associated with perimenopause. Interpersonal therapy explores the relationships in your life and how they may be contributing to your emotional problems. This type of therapy also teaches you how to use the strength and support you gain from your relationships to help deal with emotional issues. Cognitive-behavioral therapy examines your core thoughts and beliefs and how they determine your actions in response to life. If you have developed a pessimistic or negative attitude toward life in general, this type of therapy can help you see the world in a more balanced perspective and learn more effective ways of coping.

Insomnia and Its Role in Menopause

Long-term insomnia (a condition characterized by an inadequate amount or poor quality of sleep occurring three or more nights a week) can contribute to heightened anxiety and feelings of daytime fatigue, moodiness, and irritability. When women don't get enough rest, they can have difficulty with concentration, focus, and memory, and their overall physical and mental health can suffer.

With nearly 40 million people in the United States suffering from some sort of sleep disorder, it's a given that a large number of perimenopausal and menopausal women are among them. In fact, the National Sleep Foundation's (an independent, nonprofit organization) 1998 poll, Women and Sleep, found that the average woman between the ages of thirty and sixty sleeps only six hours and forty-one minutes a night during the workweek. "Women are probably the most sleep-deprived creatures on earth," according to Joyce A. Walsleben, Ph.D., director of the

Sleep Disorders Center at the New York University School of Medicine.

Good, restful sleep is essential to physical and mental well-being. Every woman approaching menopause should understand the connection between her life phase and her sleep cycles, so she can be prepared to overcome sleep problems that might develop during this time.

Hormonal Imbalances and Sleeplessness

A woman's hormonal balance affects her ability to sleep throughout her adult life; many women experience sleep disturbances during menstruation, pregnancy, and in perimenopause and menopause.

Women who experience PMS (premenstrual syndrome) often report sleeping difficulties during that same, late phase of the menstrual cycle (Days 22 through 28). Physical symptoms of PMS, such as bloating, headache, and cramping, can contribute to sleeplessness. But women with PMS report a range of sleep problems in addition to insomnia, including hypersomnia (a condition in which you sleep too much) and daytime sleepiness. As women who have a history of PMS approach menopause, those symptoms can become more severe.

Women in menopause report more sleep disorders than women in any other age group. Many sleep problems in perimenopause are caused by other symptoms of diminishing hormones, including hot flashes and night sweats. Although these problems may not be severe enough to actually cause a person to awaken, they can disrupt sleep cycles frequently enough to cause fatigue and sleepiness throughout the following day.

The Source of Sleep Problems

Remember, hormonal imbalances and insomnia can feed feelings of anxiety and depression. The less rested you are, the more powerful your negative feelings become, and the less able you are to see your way through them. Stress—an enemy of women at any age—can also severely inhibit your ability to enjoy deep, restful sleep. If you "snap" awake at four A.M. for no good reason and lie in bed worrying about vague concerns or relatively inconsequential issues until the alarm goes off at seven A.M., stress is playing a role in your sleep disturbance.

Your sleep problems may have nothing to do with stress, anxiety, or tension but could have physical sources. One in four women over fifty, for example, suffers from sleep apnea, a sleep disorder in which the sleeper stops breathing for frequent, short periods throughout the night. Snoring and daytime sleepiness are clues that you might be suffering from sleep apnea. Snoring can increase with weight gain—particularly when you gain weight around your neck. If you have a problem with daytime sleepiness and your partner complains your snoring is louder and more pronounced, see your doctor. Sleep apnea is associated with other medical problems, including high blood pressure and cardiovascular disease, so it isn't something to blow off.

Drugs Used to Treat Insomnia

Though many doctors recommend HRT for the relief of insomnia, depression, and anxiety, a number of prescription medications are available to help menopausal women combat these debilitating conditions. However, try over-the-counter sleep aids first.

More women than men suffer pain-related sleep problems. Pain from arthritis, migraine headaches, tension, chronic fatigue syndrome, and fibromyalgia have been linked to sleep disruption in women. Pain can make falling asleep and sleeping through the night more difficult, but many people fail to report (or recognize) sleeplessness as a problem. If pain is interrupting your sleep, ask your health-care professional about your pain management options.

Finally, if you're already dealing with fluctuating hormones and subsequent hot flashes, night sweats, and periodic anxiety attacks, the disruption of travel can also make your sleep problems even more severe.

Is Your Lifestyle Keeping You Awake?

Simple lifestyle choices may be at the root of many sleep disturbances. Here are some of the most common daily habits that can interfere with good, restful sleep:

- **Alcohol:** Drinking alcohol right before bedtime may help you fall asleep initially, but it's also likely to wake you up hours before you're ready to rise. Avoid alcohol for at least two to four hours before heading for bed.
- **Caffeine:** Caffeine can stimulate your brain and make it difficult to go to sleep and stay asleep. Limit the amount of caffeine you consume during the day, and confine that consumption to the morning or early afternoon hours. Or cut out the caffeine altogether by switching to decaf drinks or mineral water. Remember, it's not just coffee that contains caffeine; it is also found in colas and other "brown" sodas, nonherbal teas, and some headache medications.
- **Exercising at night:** Exercise regularly to help put your body on a natural schedule, but don't exercise in the two to three hours before bedtime.
- **Smoking:** Nicotine is a stimulant. Your good health requires that you quit altogether, but if you do continue to smoke, stop at least two to three hours before bedtime.
- **Your sleep environment:** Keep the sleeping room temperature between 65 and 70 degrees. Use light-blocking window shades or wear a sleep mask. Close the doors and windows to block out

sound; play calm, soothing music with the device set to shut off automatically. And finally, consider sleeping apart from disruptive sleep partners of any species—including pets (a difficult step, but perhaps essential).

Putting Sleep Disorders to Rest

You may think that missing an hour or two of sleep now and then isn't a problem, but you're probably wrong. If you aren't getting enough sleep—and that means at least eight hours a day for most adults—your physical and emotional health will suffer.

The most important way to promote and protect healthy sleep patterns is to pay attention to sleep problems when they arise and then take action to resolve them. If the lifestyle changes suggested in the preceding section don't alleviate your sleep problems, seek professional help. You have a number of options, including changing your diet, exercise schedule, medications, hormone replacement therapy, relaxation techniques, biofeedback, and psychological counseling.

Though sleep disturbances may be a short episode in your passage to menopause, you shouldn't allow them to get the upper hand. Insomnia, anxiety, and fatigue go hand in hand, but they don't have to grab hold of you during perimenopause and menopause. Protect your sleep, so you can protect your health.

Staying "On the Level"

If you are experiencing mild mood disturbances, anxiety, or general but recurring feelings of the blues, you have a number of simple self-treatment options for leveling out your emotional roller-coaster ride.

First, give your body and mind healthy amounts of good fuel, activity, and rest. Eat a healthy diet that emphasizes fruit, vegetables, and whole grains and skips high-fat, low-nutrient foods loaded with sugar, salt, and simple carbohydrates. Limiting caffeine, salt, MSG, and sugar can help your body remain active and alert rather than jumpy and fatigued. Your physical and emotional health are inextricably linked, and you can't maintain either with a crummy diet.

Never Self-Medicate

According to the North American Menopause Society, women are more likely than men to increase their consumption of alcohol when depressed. Abusing alcohol or drugs compounds the problems of midlife, and women in perimenopause should be wary of self-medicating with these substances. Don't borrow a friend's sleeping pills, and consult your doctor if you find yourself taking even over-the-counter sleeping aids on a more than sporadic basis.

Here are some other good guidelines to follow:

- **Eat sensible amounts of food throughout the day.** If you stuff yourself or try to eat your way out of a low mood, you just add to the problem by contributing to weight gain, low self-esteem, and poor body image. But if you skip meals or rely on junk food because you're too busy to worry about when and what you're eating, you can stress both your body and mind—and rob them of nutrients they need. If you're pressed for time, check out the frozen foods section of your grocery. Lots of frozen meals are tasty, nutritious, and low in fat and calories.
- **Be active.** Activity is one of the best ways to lift and stabilize your mood. Physical activity triggers your body to release mood-lifting endorphins, and it gets your heart pumping to circulate healthy, oxygenated blood throughout your body. Participating

in activities with family and friends can help lighten your mood, broaden your perspective on the issues that are troubling you, and renew your hopes and interests so you can deal more effectively with issues that threaten your emotional health.

- **Practice meditation or relaxation techniques.** Meditation, yoga, and t'ai chi are powerful tools for relieving hot flashes and other symptoms of stress, anxiety, and mild depression. (See Chapters 16 and 17 for more information on meditation and yoga.) Fifteen-minute sessions of meditation, deep breathing, or relaxation every morning and evening can reduce or even eliminate stress and mood-altering emotional upheavals. Prayer is a similar, more traditional way for many people to find solace.

- **Get plenty of rest.** Try to establish and maintain a regular sleep schedule: Go to sleep and rise at the same times every day—including weekends. Take time to read, listen to music, or soak in a hot tub to relax and prepare yourself for sleep. Don't exercise or eat large amounts of food late in the evening.

You Don't Have to Go It Alone

No one treatment option is right—or even effective—for every woman. But any woman suffering from mood disorders should talk with a doctor, counselor, or mentor to discuss appropriate treatments. If your usual health-care provider does not seem to have the answers, do not assume that the problem is "you"; get a second opinion. Though women are statistically more likely than men to suffer from depression, they are also more likely to look for help in overcoming issues that affect their emotional health. A willingness to admit and discuss mood disorders is your best weapon for overcoming them.

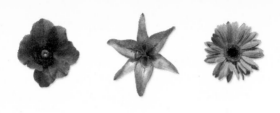

chapter eleven | *Menopause* **and Sexuality**

Women in perimenopause are often surprised to find their sexual appetites changing. The reasons for shifts in sexual readiness and desire are as complex as human sexuality itself and include physical, emotional, psychological, and chemical changes natural in a maturing body. These changes are far more complex in the older woman than in the older man. By learning more about the potential impact of menopause on your own sexuality, you're better prepared to manage your experience.

A New Sexual Revolution

If you believe that menopause equals the end of sex as you know it, you're wrong. Today, most people know that idea is simply untrue and dismiss it as outdated mythology. In fact, the American Association of Retired Persons (AARP) *Modern Maturity* Sexual Survey, conducted in 1999, showed over two-thirds of men and women age forty-five and older say they're satisfied with their sex lives, and many say they enjoy sex "now more than ever." Still, not everyone understands all of the ways the physical changes of menopause can affect sexuality.

Sex and Growing Older

A landmark 1986 study by Masters & Johnson (Sex and Aging— Expectations and Reality) found that women can remain sexually active their entire lives with no decline in orgasmic potential and may become more orgasmic. The study also found that normal changes of sexual response and aging don't equate to decreased sexual functioning.

Thanks to the burgeoning numbers of women moving into midlife today, the discussion, research, and medical information on maturing female sexuality has never been richer. Talking about libido with other people is no longer considered taboo. Women can turn to doctors, health-care professionals, and books such as this one to educate themselves about exactly what kinds of physical symptoms and changes may affect their sexuality during menopause and how to maintain optimum sexual health during this time. That understanding paves the way for a sexual revolution as socially significant as the first one these Baby Boomers experienced back in the 1960s—an era of the sexually confident, healthy, and vital midlife woman!

The Physical Facts of Life

Once you acknowledge that sexual problems of midlife aren't all in the head, the next step is understanding the physical symptoms and changes that can interfere with sexual desire and pleasure as menopause approaches. Here are the most common:

- Vaginal dryness
- Pain during penetration
- Reduced response to clitoral stimulation and other sexual stimuli

Some of these changes are absolutely normal parts of the aging process. Women (and men, for that matter) typically experience a slowdown in their biologic sexual response. Women may take longer to become aroused, for example, and some women report that they have fewer orgasmic contractions and shorter orgasms in general. These changes just mean that lovemaking takes on a new schedule or some new practices. Other physical changes are transient and treatable, either with medical hormonal therapies or nonhormonal, natural techniques.

But there are also a number of physical and medical events that can trigger the symptoms and conditions of flagging sexual health, as well. These events include:

- Illnesses, both physical and emotional, including (but not limited to) cardiac problems, hypertension, cancer, bladder disease, depression, and arthritis.
- Medications used to treat any of the above illnesses, including some antihypertensives, antidepressants, tranquilizers, and antihistamines.
- Medical treatments, such as radiation therapy, chemotherapy, or surgery.

Don't get the impression that if you take blood pressure medication or undergo surgery, you're embarking on a life of sexual abstinence. Sexual dysfunction resulting from illness or long-term treatments such as chemotherapy can pass as the illness and treatment side effects fade. A number of alternative medications can replace those that create sexual problems for certain individuals.

Hormones and Sexuality

Let's not forget diminishing estrogen levels is one of the primary causes for many sexual health issues in perimenopausal and menopausal women. Hormonal imbalances can trigger or exacerbate many of the physical symptoms that erode a healthy, perimenopausal woman's sex life.

Hormones—especially estrogen—play an important role in your body's sexual response. Estrogen helps to nourish all of your body's tissues, including your vagina, vulva, and urethra. Estrogen also helps keep the clitoris well nourished and responsive; with less estrogen, the clitoris can lose some of its ability to respond to touch.

As your vaginal wall becomes thinner and drier, your vagina can become shorter, narrower, and less elastic. If this vaginal atrophy becomes severe, sex can be quite painful. Lack of lubrication and vaginal walls that just won't give can make sex less appealing—to both the woman and her partner.

A lack of estrogen will also result in a change in the normal vaginal pH, and lower levels of lactobacillus, the normal bacteria that helps ward off most vaginal infections in reproductive-age women. Thus, if your vagina goes through marked changes in pH levels, you may find that you're more susceptible to vaginal infections, which can make your vagina feel raw and irritated, create abnormal vaginal discharge, and make sexual intercourse a painful, burning experience. Estrogen replacement therapy can improve vaginal secretions and tone and can even be used in the form of a vaginal cream, suppositories, or a synthetic ring, in order to deliver the hormone locally for more rapid effects.

Hormones play another critical role in strengthening or diminishing the libido; the sex hormones—estrogen and progesterone—contribute to mood. If you grow anxious, depressed, irritable, or exhausted as a result of hormone deficiencies, your sex life can suffer.

Beyond the Physical Factor

Without question, a woman's psychological and emotional state can trigger many physical symptoms. When a woman has low self-esteem or a poor body image, for example, she can have a greatly reduced response to stimulation. Anxiety, sleeplessness, and hot flashes can interfere with a woman's ability to anticipate or enjoy sex and contribute to one or more of the previously listed physical symptoms. Decreased sexual activity itself can lead to diminished sexual desire, pleasure, and response.

Any woman knows that her most important responses to sexual stimulation take place in her brain; as a result, any number of conditions or illnesses can impair a woman's libido, including alcoholism, fatigue, depression, and chronic illnesses. It's hard to dispute the fact that our libido is all tangled up in our self-esteem. Perimenopause and natural menopause are transitions associated with aging, and if self-esteem suffers as a result of aging, sexual desire may suffer, too.

Our bodies change during perimenopause; that, too, is an undeniable fact. The degree of that change varies, of course, and we have many tools at our disposal to help maintain our physical health and vitality as we grow older. But women who combat weight gain, fatigue, depression, and feelings of isolation during perimenopause are at risk for suffering from diminished sexual desire, as well.

Maintaining Your Sexual Health

If you, like the vast majority of men and women in this country, intend to remain sexually active throughout a long and healthy life, what can you do to ensure that you maintain your sexual health through the years ahead? Well, how do you get to Carnegie Hall? Practice, practice, practice, especially when you're by yourself. Before you begin any treatments, you have four basic tools at your disposal:

- Monitor your sexual health and pay attention to changes in your sexual responses and feelings.
- Maintain an open dialog with your health-care professional about sexual problems and solutions.
- Maintain your vaginal health.
- Use appropriate birth control methods while still in perimenopause.

Take Your Partner Along for the Ride

The most commonly reported reason for sexual dissatisfaction in older women is lack of a suitable partner. If you are lucky enough to be in a committed relationship as you near midlife (and let me tell you, then you are *really* lucky), the chances are good that your partner in that relationship is changing and aging, too. Men can experience a loss of sexual potency and desire as they age, and that can have a direct impact on the sexual confidence and health of their partners. If a sexual partner seems uninterested in sex or unable to sustain an erection or become aroused, it's easy for the other partner to feel inadequate, undesirable, and definitely unsexy.

Enjoyment Increases

In a survey of forty-five- to sixty-five-year-old men and women conducted in 2001 by *Newsweek* magazine, 30 percent of women and 34 percent of men surveyed thought sex is more enjoyable for people their age than for younger people, 40 percent of women and 47 percent of men said it was "about the same," and only 16 percent and 12 percent (respectively) thought sex "less enjoyable" with age.

Your partner's sexual performance and desire may be suffering as much—or even more—than your own. If you and your partner experience a decline in sexual intimacy, you should talk about it. Many couples ignore sexual problems because they're too embarrassed to discuss them together—let alone with a doctor or other health-care professional. But most sexual issues don't resolve themselves. Even if you take action to improve your own sexual response and desire, your partner may not benefit from your experience. In fact, some men and women can feel a bit overwhelmed by their partner's increased sexual desire. Talking with your partner is your first step to getting your sex life back on track. With talking, timing is everything. Don't address a major sexual issue right after an episode of less than satisfactory sex, when your partner can't go back in time and fix what just happened. Choose a comfortable but nonsexual setting to make a request about a change.

Explore All Your Lovemaking Options

As he ages, your male partner may need more stimulation in order to achieve an erection. As you're learning to enjoy your sexuality more, don't forget to pay attention to your partner's needs. Many couples find that as their sexual relationship matures they draw increasing pleasure from the nonintercourse parts of their lovemaking and use their hands and mouths more frequently during sex.

If your partner is suffering from physical problems that are affecting his or her sexual performance, a general practitioner or gynecologist may decide to refer you to a sex therapist. Keep an open mind and follow your doctor's recommendations. Maintaining the health of your sexual relationship is an important part of remaining healthy and happy together.

You have an important opportunity to improve your sex life during perimenopause. With the wide variety of physical and psychological tools available to you, you can take your sexuality to new heights as your body enjoys sex for reasons that have nothing to do with reproduction.

What If Your Mate Is Menopausal, Too?

Though the phenomenon of male menopause was first the subject of research in the 1940s, even twenty years ago you would have had to search for scientific references to male menopause. Today, the medical and psychological communities treat the subject with much more respect.

Problems with Impotence

Sexual dysfunction isn't the only marker of male menopause. Studies show that nearly 51 percent of men ages forty to seventy experience some level of impotence in varying degrees of severity and persistence—and that's many more than the number who exhibit symptoms of male menopause.

Many men do experience a psychosocial passage known as a midlife crisis, triggered by flagging sexuality, career plateaus, and the realization that having it all isn't all it was cracked up to be. But that midlife event, as important as it may be, isn't the same as male menopause.

Male menopause, known as *andropause* to the medical community, affects (by some reports) nearly 40 percent of men between the ages of forty and sixty. All men begin producing less testosterone after the age of forty. As testosterone levels decrease, men may find that they experience fewer erections, that the erections are less easy to sustain, and that they experience longer intervals between erections. Male menopause can result in a wide range of symptoms in men, including lethargy, depression, mood swings, insomnia, hot flashes, irritability, and decreased sexual desire.

Diminishing testosterone in the bloodstream isn't the only culprit behind male menopause. Other factors include obesity, excess alcohol consumption, hypertension and the medications used to treat it, lack of exercise, and other "middle-age plagues" that damage health. While medications have been developed to treat erectile dysfunction, testosterone therapy is one of the few nonbehavioral medical treatments available for combating male menopause.

Two Women in Menopause

If you are in a same-sex relationship, the chances are very good that at some point you and your mate may both be experiencing symptoms of approaching menopause. Although it may seem that sharing a household with another menopausal woman could lead to increased conflict, you also have a life-partner who may be better able to understand your experience. Both of you will need to remember, however, that every woman's menopause experience is unique, so neither of you can expect the other to have the same symptoms or reactions to those symptoms.

So what does this have to do with your passage through perimenopause and menopause?

If you and your mate are both experiencing the mood swings, irritability, and other negative effects of menopause at the same time, both of you may have a rougher time dealing with the experience. Two women going through perimenopause at the same time may experience a multitude of sexual issues as they try to maintain their sexual closeness while each rides her own roller coaster of menopausal symptoms.

What It All Means for You

The bottom line is, your partner may or may not understand or accept his or her own struggle with midlife passage, and that could put extra demands on your patience and understanding—at a time when you won't feel particularly well-endowed with either. Your partner may not have the reserves of patience and support necessary to help you through all of the rough patches of menopause, and at times you may have to draw on your deepest supply of those qualities to avoid throwing gasoline on the smoldering fires of family discord.

Listen to Your Sexual Self

One of the most important things you can do to maintain your sexual health is to pay attention to what your body and mind are telling you about your feelings regarding your sexuality, your attitude toward sex in general, and your evolving sexual response. Your sexuality evolves with the rest of you, and the entire package has changed dramatically over the past twenty years. Changing interests and attitudes aren't a sign of age—they're a sign of maturity. If you always enjoyed romantic, sexy actors in films and don't find that Leonardo di Caprio does anything for you right now, don't despair: Think more toward the lines of Sean Connery or Mel Gibson. As your sexual tastes evolve, you can find totally new and different ways to enjoy sex, and that's just one of the benefits of seniority.

But if you suddenly realize that sex no longer holds any interest for you; or that you don't like your body enough to share it in sexual relations with anyone; or that it's just too painful, awkward, difficult, or otherwise unpleasant to "mess with" sex, you need to stop and ask yourself when—and why—these feelings arose in you.

Remember, the old saying "use it or lose it" is frequently applied to sexuality. Long periods of abstinence can undermine your ability to become aroused, and lack of sexual activity can promote vaginal atrophy and a diminished response to sexual stimulation.

You deserve and benefit from a healthy, active sexual self—whether you have a partner or not. If you aren't enjoying (or even thinking about) sex, you have many options for regaining your sexual enjoyment—whether that involves exploring new sexual techniques, examining your attitudes about your sexuality, or investigating possible medical causes for your diminishing sexual interests or abilities.

Stay Healthy

The primary physical component of an active, healthy sexuality is a healthy vagina. Your vagina is maturing along with the rest of your body, and it's worth your while to pay attention to caring for this sensitive (and vital) part of your body.

First, if your sexual life involves new partners, always practice safe sex. This isn't the 1960s, and casual, unprotected sex with strangers never again will be in fashion. Don't count on your judgment or gut reaction to determine whether or not someone's infected with AIDS or other sexually transmitted diseases (STDs). Assume that they are—no matter who they are—and don't allow a sexual partner's semen, blood, or other body fluids to come in contact with your vagina, anus, or mouth. Your vaginal tissues are becoming thinner and easier to tear, and your immune system might be stressed by shifting hormone levels. That puts you more at risk than ever for contracting a sexually transmitted disease. Talk to your partner about his or her sexual history, use condoms, and get blood tests. Safe sex practices may not seem sexy, but they're basic to survival.

Don't Forget about Birth Control

Remember, until you have gone for twelve months without a period or until your doctor or health-care provider has run appropriate blood tests to determine the levels of hormones your body is producing, you could ovulate and, therefore, become pregnant. A surprise pregnancy in your mid-forties can be a tremendous problem for both you and your partner. Be smart, and use contraceptives for a year after your last period.

Next, take steps to reduce vaginal dryness. Estrogen replacement is one way to combat vaginal dryness, but over-the-counter vaginal moisturizers such as Astroglide, K-Y Jelly, and Vagisil Moisturizer can help fight off dryness, too, especially when caused by additional friction during intercourse.

Avoid vaginal deodorizers and deodorized products, scented toilet tissues, and chemical-laden bath soaps and soaks. Perfumes and chemicals can further upset the pH balance in your vagina and contribute to local irritation and dryness. Be sure to drink plenty of water and eat a diet rich in fruit, whole grains, and vegetables.

Check Your Sexual Attitude

Your age and hormone levels don't determine your sexuality; you are who you have always been, and your fundamental feelings and attitudes about sex don't change when you stop ovulating. But the physical and emotional evolution of a maturing mind and body can color your sexual response.

Take a Multivitamin

A multivitamin-mineral supplement may be an easy and inexpensive way to promote your sexuality—and your general health. Vitamin E has been shown in some studies to increase sexual desire, and zinc may help foster sexual arousal (oysters are high in zinc).

Selenium is another mineral that is the subject of ongoing studies of sexuality, as is L-carnitine. Both are available as over-the-counter supplements.

Your attitudes about sex and your own sexuality today are greatly influenced by the attitudes you had about these issues when you were younger. If you enjoyed sex and expected to be sexually satisfied when you were thirty, you're more likely to continue to enjoy sex as you move through your fifties and beyond.

Every woman has unique sexual needs and interests, and many women (and men) have a limited sexual desire at some point in their lives. But if you find your interest in sex waning—at any age—it's important for you to understand why. Maintaining and nurturing your sexuality is important for your physical and emotional health.

Your ability to talk about issues—ranging from painful intercourse to a lack of response to stimulation—is crucial to establish a trusting relationship with your health-care provider. If sex is physically less enjoyable—even painful—your gynecologist, internist, or other health-care provider can prescribe medications, exercises, or other treatments. A professional counselor or therapist can also help if a lack of interest in sex is a side effect of a growing sense of depression and isolation.

Overcoming Physical Barriers

If you don't feel physically fit and healthy, you're less likely to enjoy an active, healthy sex life. Although you can't postpone menopause or the effects of aging indefinitely, the physical symptoms of menopause shouldn't prevent you from remaining sexually active. As mentioned above, talking with your gynecologist or other health-care provider about treatments will help. You may also be able to improve your sexual health through some changes in your lifestyle choices.

The Basics

The same stresses, habits, and substances that damage other aspects of your health can limit your desire and ability to enjoy sex, as well. Remember these basics for maintaining your sexual fitness:

- **Eat right and exercise regularly:** Regular aerobic, weight-bearing, and stretching exercises keep your body feeling active and alive. Middle-age weight gain and ebbing muscle strength and endurance can erode your sexual desire. When your body is strong and fit, you're more energetic and you take a greater interest in all aspects of your life—including sex. Plus, exercise releases endorphins, the "feel happy" neurotransmitters in your brain. If you feel better about your body, you're more likely to feel good about sharing it with someone physically.

The Exercise Boost

Exercise offers a number of benefits for women at any age, but did you know that it could give you a real sexual boost? Some studies have shown that people who practice some form of regular exercise achieve orgasm more easily than do people who don't exercise at all.

- **Rest and manage stress:** Stress can lead to headaches, indigestion, muscle pain, depression, and—not surprisingly—a diminished desire for and response to sexual activity. If your daily routine is too overwhelming to allow you to enjoy an active sex life, it's probably damaging your health in other ways. Learn what's causing your stress, then do what you can to avoid the stressors.

- **Cut down on alcohol and stop smoking:** Drinking too much alcohol can lead to depression, weight gain, and—in some cases—an increased stress response. Smoking fuels stress, and it saps your body of strength and energy. All of these effects can erode your interest in sexual activity and dampen your response to sexual stimulation.

- **Treat vaginal dryness:** As mentioned earlier, estrogen replacement can help relieve vaginal dryness and keep vaginal tissues moist, elastic, and healthy. Women who cannot use estrogen replacement therapy now have newer options, such as estrogen suppositories (one brand is Vagifem) that act only in the vagina. Because it is not absorbed into the woman's general circulation, it does not increase the risk of a recurrence of breast cancer or other estrogen-sensitive conditions.

Do Something Different!

Don't become complacent about your sex life. Set the right mood, and if you've stopped paying attention to your physical appearance, take some time to do the things that will make you look and feel more beautiful. Get a new haircut or have a facial. Stop by the cosmetics counter at your local department store, and ask for some ideas for revitalizing your appearance. Buy a sexy new bra or nightgown: Styles are available for women of all shapes and sizes. Some women even choose to leave their sexy new lingerie or peignoir on, while making love, to cover any troublesome areas or old surgical scars. When you look better to yourself, you feel more sexually appealing.

Enjoy Your Body

If you lead a hectic life, filled with the responsibilities of work, home, and family, you may have little time to think about yourself—your body, your mind, your pleasure.

The truth is, your body matters, and your physical needs matter, too. If you find yourself looking at your body with disappointment or wanting to ignore your body and its physical condition and needs, take conscious action to overcome those feelings. Your body is yours for life, and keeping it healthy and fit is vital as you approach menopause.

Spending time caring for your body will encourage you to take pleasure in its strength and capabilities. By feeling confident and at ease about your body, you're more likely to enjoy the pleasures of its sexual responses. Learn to include your sexuality in your self-identity; humans are sexual beings, and sexual enjoyment is good for both the body and the mind.

Explore your sexual interests and fantasies. Don't feel ashamed of your sexual orientation, desires, or needs. Many doctors and sex therapists encourage their patients to masturbate to increase their ability to respond to sexual stimulation and to combat stress and anxiety. By experimenting in private, you should be able to tell your partner what makes you feel good more easily. If you'd like more information on how to become aroused and stay stimulated (by yourself or with a partner), visit your local bookstore, which is full of self-help books on improving your sexual response. Even reading a steamy novel can help you to become aroused. Or rent a film with some love scenes featuring a favorite movie star. You don't have to turn to pornography, just allow yourself to explore and enjoy the sexual arousal you might normally hold back.

Enhancing Your Sexual Experience

If your lovemaking simply needs some new life, take this opportunity to enjoy a second "first romance" with your partner. Schedule an actual "date"; prepare for it by buying some aromatherapy candles or new pillowcases—this may help you get in the mood, too. Learn to touch each other again and take pleasure in your physical contact; take baths and showers together and spend more time in touching and foreplay during lovemaking. Let your partner know what feels good to you, find out what he or she enjoys most, and explore your fantasies. Don't forget to use vaginal creams and lubricants to make the sexual experience more enjoyable. (If you're using condoms, remember to use water-based lubricants; petroleum can weaken the condom wall and cause breaks and tears.) Your bodies are yours to enjoy, so don't hold back.

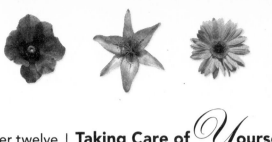

chapter twelve | **Taking Care of *Yourself***

It's true that the human body becomes more susceptible to certain diseases and conditions with age and that women face special health concerns as their natural hormone supply diminishes in menopause. As you move through midlife and approach menopause, there is some good news about aging, however. When it comes to longevity, women have a decided advantage over men—despite the many physical changes they will undergo during their lifetime. On average, women live about six years longer than men and hold this advantage in life expectancy throughout the life cycle. (In a 2000 report, The U.S. Census Bureau projected that the average life expectancy for men as 74, versus 80 for women.) This decided difference in life expectancy between men and women is expected to grow wider until around 2050, when it finally levels off.

Health experts have debated the reasons why women tend to live longer than men for years. Some have speculated that women are just hardier creatures. Others have attributed the difference to the fact that men, on average, were exposed to more environmental hazards than women, but this is changing as more females become firefighters, enlist in the Marines, take the bus to work every day, and so on. Let's take a quick look at some of the most current hypotheses on the issue.

- **Sex-linked differences:** One school of thought suggests that women at all ages have stronger immune resistance and are additionally protected from certain health problems by female hormones such as estrogen.

- **Differences in health habits:** Women, in general, tend to take better care of their health and avoid potentially harmful habits such as cigarette smoking and excessive alcohol consumption. This isn't to say, however, that smoking is no longer a health issue among women. Recent studies by the U.S. Department of Health and Human Services have shown that smoking rates are gradually increasing among young women despite health warnings and education efforts. (As mentioned previously, if you smoke, now is the time to quit. If you quit now, you'll be an excellent role model for your teenage daughters or granddaughters, in case they are toying with the habit without realizing its addictive potential.)

However, many women tend to forget about or ignore their special dietary requirements and, in so doing, place their health in jeopardy and adversely affect their potential longevity. In Chapter 13, you'll learn more about eating healthfully and about some of the most important nutrients for women.

Appreciate Your Changing Body

Proper nutrition is not the only thing women sometimes forget about. At a time when life is increasingly hectic for women experiencing perimenopause, it's easy to neglect taking care of yourself in other ways. You are more than a pair of breasts, a uterus, a heart, and a set of bones; you're a woman, with a life full of interests that extend well beyond disease prevention.

Every woman expects the natural changes of age to occur, but in a culture that seems to worship the physical impossibilities of eternal youth, rail-like thinness, and nonstop sexual vigor and allure, maintaining an appreciation and respect for your body as it ages can be difficult. One of the benefits of maturity is a growing appreciation for the valuable things pop culture often fails to acknowledge. If you continue to evaluate your appearance and physical capabilities in comparison to those of a twenty-year-old, you're destined to be dissatisfied and disappointed.

Reality Check

According to the National Center for Health Statistics, the average woman in the United States over the age of twenty is just under 5'4" tall and weighs 152 pounds. Some studies of women in the fashion industry reveal that the average fashion model is 5'11" tall and weighs 117 pounds. You can decide for yourself which of these is more realistic.

Acknowledge and appreciate the woman you are now. Then, focus your attention on keeping that woman as healthy and happy as you possibly can. If you feel better, you'll look better. Taking good care of the woman you are today is the first and most important secret to looking and feeling your best through menopause and beyond.

Taking Care of Your Changing Body

You depend upon your senses to remain in communication with the world around you, and good eyesight and hearing are essential to that dialog. Though few women need to worry about experiencing a rapid decline in the quality of their vision or hearing as they near the age of menopause, those functions can begin to diminish around the age of forty or fifty. Some of the physical changes of menopause can have an impact on the health of your skin, hair and teeth, as well. Though age-related changes are inevitable, you can minimize their impact by taking special care of your skin, hair, teeth, eyes, and ears; by watching for signs and symptoms of potential problems; and by incorporating regular checkups into your regular health-care routine. Prevention is easier than treatment—and cheaper, too.

Taking Care of Your Changing Mind

Most medical and scientific authorities agree that the mind's ability to think clearly and quickly changes with age, but those changes aren't linked to menopause. Changes in the brain's physical size and functions occur with age, and those changes can have an impact on how well you can recall information stored in your brain.

Perhaps most important to preserving memory and recall is the brain's hippocampus—the part of the brain where memory is stored, created, and retrieved. It may also be the part of the brain that is integral for libido. With age, metabolic changes and a dwindling number of dendrites—the neurons that transmit the brain's signals—can exacerbate the brain's slowdown. All of these changes can combine to make your brain feel duller and slower. The information is all there and your brain can retrieve it—that retrieval process just takes longer than it used to.

Bust Stress

Physical exercise is a great way to reduce stress, and stress can take a serious toll on cognitive functions. Stress inhibits your ability to concentrate and it can shorten your lifespan. The New

England Centenarian Study has found that one trait common among those who live beyond the age of one hundred is an ability to handle stress.

You don't need to panic that you're suffering an onset of early Alzheimer's disease every time you misplace your car keys. Many of the symptoms of menopause, including mood swings, sleeplessness, and fluctuating levels of hormones, can contribute to less efficient cognitive functions. Later in this chapter, you'll learn some practical methods for combating memory loss.

Monitoring Changes in Vision

Around the age of forty, many women begin to experience ocular problems, otherwise known as changes in vision. The shape of your eyeball can change as you age, and the subsequent reduction of your visual acuity can be subtle at first. A few of the most common problems you might encounter after age forty include:

- Having difficulty reading small print or seeing objects that are close to your eyes clearly. This condition is known as presbyopia and usually is easy to correct with reading glasses or even over-the-counter magnifying glasses from the drugstore.
- Noticing tiny specks or odd dustlike particles passing before your vision. These "floaters" usually are just a normal condition of the aging eye. If they become extreme in number or are accompanied by bright flashes of light, you should contact your ophthalmologist immediately. A sudden increase in the numbers of floaters can be a warning of a retinal tear or other more serious vision problem.

- Experiencing difficulties with your eyes becoming dry and irritated after you spend some time reading or working at the computer. Again, this problem isn't unusual in over-forty eyes, and you may be able to alleviate it by using "artificial tears" (available over the counter in most drugstores) for better lubrication.

Pay attention to your vision; don't ignore developing problems. All women (and men for that matter) after the age of forty should get regular annual eye examinations by an ophthalmologist. Women over the age of fifty are at particular risk of developing eye diseases, some of which might be connected to the loss of the body's natural estrogens. Your ophthalmologist will check for the following age-related diseases during your exam:

- **Macular degeneration** attacks the center of the retina, so central vision diminishes while peripheral vision remains unchanged. Macular degeneration can make reading and driving impossible; it's the number-one cause of blindness in women age sixty-five and over. No cure for the disease is known, but its risk factors include being menopausal or postmenopausal, a family history of the disease, smoking, perhaps high blood pressure, and overexposure to the sun and other ultraviolet (UV) rays. Some studies, such as the Beaver Dam Study in 2000, suggested that estrogen replacement helps postpone or prevent the onset of macular degeneration; talk to your doctor for more information.
- **Glaucoma** damages the optic nerve and is caused by a buildup of fluid, and thus pressure, inside the eye. When doctors detect and treat glaucoma early, the eye can escape permanent nerve damage. Chronic glaucoma develops slowly and, in most cases, is only detectable in its early stage through an eye examination.

Acute glaucoma can happen suddenly, blurring the vision and causing a number of symptoms including nausea and dizziness. Risk factors include being over forty, being African American, having a family history of glaucoma, having diabetes, or being nearsighted. You can't guess on this based on symptoms; your doctor has to take special pressure measurements with his or her office equipment.

Medication Affects Your Eyes

Some medications can change your vision, either by reducing your ability to focus or by reducing your eyes' lubrication, making them dry and itchy. If you notice changes in your vision shortly after you've begun taking a new medication, contact the doctor who prescribed the medication and report the change immediately.

Aside from getting annual eye examinations and reporting any changes in vision to your opthamologist, eating a healthy diet and wearing good UV-resistant eye protection, i.e., sunglasses with protective lenses, while outdoors will help you to maintain good eye health.

Protecting Your Hearing

After age fifty, many women experience some hearing loss and by age sixty-five, nearly one-third of all women have some decline in hearing. Most age-related hearing loss is gradual and can develop slowly over a period of years.

Some types of hearing loss result from many years of listening to music that is too loud, a physical injury, an infection, medication, or the development of growths or tumors. These hearing losses are called sensorineural (caused by damage to the nerves that transmit sound from the ear to the brain), because the sensors in the inner ear lose their ability to send sound signals to the brain. If you spent the 1960s with your ears glued to the loud speakers at rock concerts, you could experience this type of hearing loss.

Save Your Ears

Working near loud machinery, including lawn mowers and leaf blowers, can cause serious harm to your hearing. Avoid loud noise when you can. When you can't avoid the noise, wear earplugs or protective headphones. You may feel like an old fogey when you move to the back of the rock concert crowd, but there's nothing young and sexy about losing your hearing or having to wear a hearing-aid later in life.

Conductive hearing loss occurs when sounds don't reach your inner ear properly, due to problems with something other than the transmitting nerves themselves. If you have a history of ear infections, damage to your eardrum, or even accumulations of earwax within your ear canal, you can experience this type of hearing loss. And, as the tissue within the ear canal becomes thinner and drier, it becomes less effective at transmitting sound. When in doubt, see an ENT (Ear, Nose, Throat) specialist, especially if your symptoms are long-term.

Regular hearing checkups can reveal either type of hearing damage, but you also need to pay attention to changes in your hearing. If you notice that you're turning the television up louder these days or constantly asking people to repeat what they've just said to you, you're probably experiencing some hearing damage. Losing your hearing can make you feel isolated and out of touch with the world around you. Take steps to protect your ears and monitor changes so you can correct problems before they become irreversible.

Keeping Your Teeth Healthy

You know about the importance of regular dental checkups, brushing, and flossing. And you also know that maintaining a healthy diet that includes a wide variety of fruit, vegetables, whole grains, and necessary vitamin and mineral supplements is an essential part of maintaining full physical health, including healthy teeth and gums. But did you know that menopause can present some special challenges to your dental health? As your body's natural estrogen supply diminishes in menopause, your gum tissues can become thinner and less elastic, and bone loss can contribute to the development of gingivitis and periodontitis—gum diseases in which the soft tissue of the jaw deteriorates around the roots of the teeth.

If the bone density of the jaw itself diminishes, the socket of the tooth loosens its grip, and tooth loss can result. Greater numbers of dentists are noticing loose teeth in their menopausal patients as the first overt sign of decreasing bone density in the body overall.

Some estimates show that over one-third of all women over the age of sixty have lost most or all of their teeth. To avoid joining that group, here's a simple plan for maintaining your dental health after forty:

- See your dentist twice a year for checkups and cleaning; more frequently if you have had problems in the past.
- Brush your teeth at least twice a day; use a recommended toothbrush and floss afterward.
- Brush for two to five minutes, morning and evening (a third cleaning after lunch would be even better)—according to the Chicago Dental Society, it takes at least two minutes of brushing to remove plaque and bacteria.
- Make sure you're getting enough calcium in your diet, and limit sugar consumption.

- Pay attention to signs of gum disease, such as bleeding or inflamed gums.
- Drink plenty of water—thirty-two to sixty-four ounces every day. Water is essential for hydrating your system. It can help rinse bacteria from your gum tissue and keep the tissue moist and healthy.

If you have the time to floss only once a day, do it at night, right before you go to sleep. That's also a good time to use anti-plaque or fluoride rinses afterwards; you'll have a six- to eight-hour period without eating or drinking, so you can absorb protective fluoride and antibacterial agents.

Caring for Your Skin and Hair

As skin ages, it loses elasticity and becomes thinner, drier, and more prone to itching and sagging. Your hair becomes thinner, too; it breaks more easily and grows in more slowly. Some of these changes are due to the body's diminishing levels of estrogen. Estrogen helps keep healthy tissues well nourished and moisturized; without it, both skin and hair lose strength and elasticity and grow thinner. Other changes are the result of age; as you grow older, your body slows in its production of new cells, and collagen production slows. Collagen is the basic bridgework, or support system, for all the fibrous tissue of your body, of which skin is only one component. Normal collagen helps keep the skin plump and resilient, providing part of the skin's support structure. Taking estrogen helps maintain the proper collagen content in tissues throughout your body.

Exposure to the sun is another culprit in the deterioration of your skin's elasticity and moisture. Ultraviolet rays begin damaging the skin of young children; as sun exposure builds over the years, the damage becomes increasingly severe and apparent. Proper use of sunscreen with enough UV protection (SPF 15 or higher) and using hats or caps and sunglasses to shade your face and eyes may delay or prevent this damage.

Skin Care Basics

Your diet, the amount of rest you get every day, the level of stress you're subjected to, and the types of pollutants that exist in your environment all play a role in the health and vitality of your skin. Women in the United States spend millions of dollars every year on skin-rejuvenating treatments like chemical peels, dermabrasion, Botox, collagen injections, and even cosmetic surgery.

All of these treatment options can improve the appearance of aging skin, but some of them are expensive and temporary. And—as with any medical treatment—all of these techniques carry some risks, which although infrequent, can include scarring and skin discoloration.

If you prefer to pursue less invasive techniques for keeping your skin looking healthy and vital, you have many options to choose from. Though your skin is unique, most women need to moisturize their skin more frequently after age forty. A number of creams, lotions, and even some prescription drugs are available today for nourishing and healing aging skin:

- Creams and lotions containing alpha hydroxy acids (AHAs) dissolve the upper layer of skin that has suffered the most damage to reveal fresher, plumper skin beneath. These products won't eliminate deep wrinkles or age spots, but they can make the skin look and feel fresher. Because some women experience skin rashes and irritations, those with sensitive skin or rosacea should not use these products without the advice of a health-care professional.

- Oils, creams, and lotions containing antioxidants and vitamin derivatives may help protect collagen, moisturize the skin's upper layer, and help diminish the visible signs of fine wrinkles. Vitamins C, E, and A are typical antioxidants used in these products.
- Retinol, a vitamin A derivative, is another common anti-aging formula component. Prescription drugs Retin-A and Renova are marketed to reduce fine-line wrinkles, build collagen, and help fade age spots.

As with any skin care products, some women report that these creams and drugs help their skin look younger and fresher, but results vary. Talk to your dermatologist to learn more.

Beyond skin-care formulas, however, you have some very basic tools at your disposal for protecting your skin. No matter what other skin care treatments you use, drinking enough water, quitting smoking, wearing sunscreen with SPF 15 or higher, and maintaining a gentle, daily skincare routine that uses mild soap and moisturizer will protect your skin and help keep it looking its best.

Keeping Your Hair Healthy and Strong

The changes in your hair growth and health postmenopause can seem downright unfair; the hair on your scalp starts to become thin, sparse, and gray, while some of the previously fine, pale hairs on your face grow thicker and darker. You can tweeze, wax, or chemically dissolve unwanted facial hair, or use electrolysis to permanently destroy the hair follicle. (Some women experience skin irritation from electrolysis.) Though some of these changes are inevitable with age, you have a number of options available to you for preserving the health and vitality of your hair.

First, the basics: Keep your hair trimmed to remove split, brittle ends and encourage volume. Some color treatments can give the effect of fullness and volumizing shampoos can coat thin hair to give it extra body. When you shampoo, use warm—not hot—water, and limit blow-drying as much as possible. Some deep conditioning treatments, used every few weeks, can help keep hair strong and less prone to breaking and splitting.

Your hair reflects your nutrition, too. Don't forget to include a wide variety of fresh fruit and vegetables in your diet, and take vitamin supplements. Proper hydration is also essential to healthy hair.

Your Health and Your Hair

Thinning, dry, brittle hair may be more than a natural sign of age. Some medications and certain systemic illnesses, such as a thyroid disorder, can also cause hair to lose its strength and vitality—even to the point of causing dramatic hair loss. Talk to your doctor or health-care provider about noticeable changes to your hair's strength and appearance; don't assume you're just looking your age.

Some prescription drugs are available to help manage menopausal hair problems:

- **Minoxidil** (marketed under the name Rogaine) works to stimulate hair follicles that may have grown dormant. Minoxidil can help restore lost hair by 10 percent or more, according to some estimates.
- **Eflornithine** may help stop unwanted hair by inhibiting the production of an enzyme that contributes to hair growth. Eflornithine (marketed in its topical form as Vaniqa) can be applied as a cream directly to the area where unwanted hair grows.

These hair and skin preparations and prescriptions take weeks, if not months, to show a result. Don't be discouraged and give up your treatment program if you don't see results overnight.

Nutrition for Your Brain

Your brain needs fuel in order to function. Some experts estimate that the brain uses 20 percent or more of the body's energy. Glucose and antioxidants are important components of your brain's nutrition, so make sure your diet includes plenty of whole grains, fruit, and vegetables. The brain also may benefit from folates—found in leafy green vegetables, lentils, and other legumes. Folic acid, a laboratory produced version of folate, is included in many multivitamins and some fortified foods. Many studies also show that daily recommended doses of vitamin E and selenium may help slow the diminishment of cognitive functions. Recently, Lipoic acid and Coenzyme Q have been recognized to improve brain health, cognitive function, and memory.

Eliminate Distractions

When you're trying to memorize or recall something important, eliminate all other distractions. Turn off the television, lower the volume on the stereo, and get to a quiet place where people aren't chattering around you. You'll find you have to put in less time and effort if you are able to concentrate better, and you'll retain the information longer.

Doctors have found that estrogen helps the brain with remembering and storing new information, so estrogen therapy can help postpone a decline in cognitive functions and protect short-term and long-term memory. Estrogen also helps improve the circulation to the brain by directly dilating the critical blood vessels involved. If you are taking estrogen therapy or HRT, you can add this benefit to the many others you'll receive.

Exercise Your Body to Keep Your Brain Healthy

Exercising at least twenty minutes a day (thirty minutes to an hour daily is best) is one great way to preserve your mental acuity. Aerobic exercise helps get the blood coursing through your system, carrying oxygen and glucose to your brain—two substances the brain needs in order to function.

Though studies are still underway to establish the link between exercise and increased brain neurons, many researchers—including those researching Alzheimer's disease—are studying the protective effects of regular physical exercise on the brain's neural paths for transmitting signals.

Exercise Your Brain to Keep It Lively

Mental exercise can increase the size of different areas of the brain, just as physical exercise increases muscle size. If you want to improve your memory, you have to make some effort to pump it up. Here are some basic brain-building practices:

- **Pay attention to what is being said and what is happening around you:** Many researchers believe that inattentiveness is a major cause of forgetfulness in people of any age. If you don't really listen and observe, your brain has no opportunity to absorb and store information. Pay attention to your own actions as well.
- **Slow down and repeat information:** When you hear a new name

or have to commit a list of things to memory, stop, slow down, and repeat the information several times. If you've just met someone, repeat that person's name during the conversation.

- **Write it down:** Keep a notepad and pen in handy places around the house—next to every telephone, by the front door, and in your car—so you can write down spur-of-the-moment ideas. Write out lists of important things to do, and read the list out loud as you think about each item and visualize some image or action that each represents to you.

- **Keep thinking:** Every day, participate in some mental activity that requires your brain to remember, reason, and react quickly. Work a crossword puzzle; play a word game, cards, or chess; debate politics with your partner; draw, paint, or play a musical instrument; take a class at the local university or adult learning center; write in a journal; or memorize a car's license plate number in the morning, then see if you still know it in the afternoon. The more you exercise your brain's ability to think, the better it will function.

Enhance Your Memory

The simple techniques offered here can give you a leg up in bolstering your ability to learn and recall new information.

Don't Numb Your Mind

Watch out for alcohol and other mind-numbing drugs. Most experts agree that a drink a day isn't health threatening, but drinking too much can deaden your brain's ability to retain and recall information. Abuse of alcohol or recreational drugs can diminish your ability to absorb stimuli from the world around you and result in a limited ability to form new memories.

Events, ideas, information that pass into the hippocampus will pass right on out again unless you do something to lock them down—by associating them with other memories already safely stored and ready for retrieval. The more associations the memory is tied to, the more likely you are to be able to store and retrieve it later. In psychology, this technique of associating new information with a range of memories for stronger recall is called elaborative encoding. It takes place in your frontal lobes—an area of your brain that can always use a good workout. Over time, people have used a number of memory devices to aid this process:

- **Create mental pictographs or visualizations:** To remember six items you must pick up at the store on the way home, you may create a mental image.
- **Use the "Roman Room":** Ancient Romans used this practice to help them memorize long speeches, lists of objects, city names, and so on. To try it, envision a room. Then place around the room visual cues that remind you of items from your to-do list, shopping list, or other types of information. Make the images vivid and compelling. Each of the room's furnishings should be a reminder of the things, people, or events you want to lock in your memory.
- **Go into training for long-term lockdown:** Review information you need to remember at least three times a day for three to five days ahead of time. At the end of this mental training, you should have the information safely in the vault.

Work hard at preserving and building your cognitive functions, and try to enjoy the ride. After all, if you're worried about your memory, you probably aren't too far down the forgetfulness trail to get your ability to store and recall new information back up to speed.

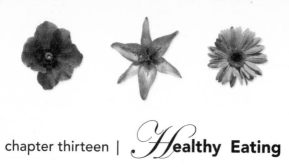

chapter thirteen | *Healthy* Eating

A healthy diet, supplemented with recommended vitamins and minerals, is your best tool for controlling or preventing some of the most damaging and debilitating conditions that affect women during and after menopause. A woman's body goes through significant changes as it approaches menopause; estrogen production slows dramatically, muscle mass decreases as fat deposits increase, metabolism slows down, body tissues—including those of the heart and circulatory system—lose elasticity, and bone cells are reabsorbed at a faster rate than they are produced. On top of that, there's the stiff, aching joints; mood swings; feelings of lethargy; and insomnia that potentially accompany menopause. All of these symptoms contribute to serious health risks stemming from two oddly disparate yet closely linked conditions—overweight and undernourishment.

The health risks of perimenopause and menopause include an increased risk of cardiovascular disease, diabetes, and osteoporosis. Add to these risks the serious health problems associated with obesity, and the challenges of maintaining your health as you approach menopause become painfully clear. Meeting these challenges requires a diet designed to both manage weight and boost nutrition.

Your Nutritional Needs after Age Forty

Many people go through life using their diets for everything but nutrition. They try one fad diet after another to lose weight; they load up on junk food and high-fat ice cream and chocolate as "food therapy" for overcoming anger, sadness, and disappointment; they choose foods based on convenience, portability, and easy cleanup. Though you may get by eating a shabby diet for a while, some time around your early forties, you might begin to feel the negative impact of bad eating habits. And even if you've always maintained a relatively healthy diet, you still may not be giving your changing body the nutrition it needs now.

What are the nutritional needs of women during and after menopause? Nutrition experts from the Institute of Medicine recommend these daily amounts of vitamins and minerals:

Nutrient (unit)	Daily Amount
Calcium (mg)	1,500 (1,200 with HRT)
Magnesium (mg/d)	320
Iron (mg/d)	5
Zinc (mg/d)	8
Iodine (mg/d)	150
Selenium (mg/d)	55
Vitamin A (mg/d)	700
Vitamin E (mg/d)	15
Vitamin D (mg/d)	10
Vitamin K (mg/d)	90
Vitamin C (mg/d)	75
Riboflavin (mg/d)	1.1
Thiamine (mg/d)	1.1
Niacin (mg/d)	14
Vitamin B_6 (mg/d)	1.5
Folate (mg/d)	400
Vitamin B_{12} (mg/d)	2.4

Table taken from the American College of Obstetricians and Gynecologists patient education publication AP151, *A Healthy Diet*.

Nutritional Boosts for Women over Forty

The following list includes some special nutritional concerns for women at the age of menopause (remember these amounts are general recommendations; women taking certain medications or combating specific conditions may need to take more or less, depending upon their doctor or health-care professional's recommendations).

- Women need to be particularly careful to consume the recommended amount of calcium every day because of the risk of developing osteoporosis. If you're postmenopausal and taking HRT, you should consume 1,200 mg daily; if you're not taking HRT, and for all women sixty-five years of age or over, 1,500 mg is a must. Calcium is in milk, yogurt, cheese, and other dairy products, as well as in fortified fruit juices. Most women need to use supplements to get the full recommended amount, without adding too many calories to your diet in the form of dairy products. One serving of dairy usually has 250 to 300 mg; learn to read labels.

- Vitamin D is an essential partner to the calcium in your diet. Your body absorbs vitamin D from the sun; if you live in a cold or northern climate or don't spend much time outdoors, vitamin D added to your calcium supplement will help your gastrointestinal system absorb the calcium. You can get 100 of the 400 IU recommended daily amount in one eight-ounce glass of skim milk. Eggs and some fish, including sardines, mackerel, and herring, contain small amounts of vitamin D, and some juices and certain brands of calcium supplements are also available with added vitamin D.

- Fiber is an important part of every woman's diet, particularly for women reaching menopause. Women should eat 25 to 30 grams of fiber daily. Soluble fiber, found in fruit, vegetables, dried beans, barley, and oats, helps keep cholesterol levels low and can help prevent heart disease and lower the risk of stroke. Insoluble fiber, found in complex carbohydrates such as whole grains and the skins of fruits and vegetables, provides bulk to keep your digestive system on track and can help prevent colon cancer.

- Antioxidants, including vitamins A, C, E, and beta carotene, are vitamins found in a number of brightly colored fruits and vegetables. These are considered important tools in warding off heart disease and some cancers and may even reduce macular degeneration (age-related vision loss). Antioxidants work to stop the effects of oxidation within your body by protecting your body tissue from the effect of free radicals—molecules in your body that lack an electron and therefore "steal" one from other body cells. Like rust-proofing treatments for your car, antioxidants block these free radicals from damaging your body's tissues. Squash, sweet potatoes, spinach, mangos, tomatoes, red peppers, oranges, blueberries, and peaches are just some of the fresh fruit and vegetable sources of antioxidants. Chocolate may also provide some antioxidant benefits, but don't forget about calories.

- Soy and other phytoestrogens can have a beneficial effect on your body as its natural hormone production slows down. Even though phytoestrogens are dramatically less potent than the body's natural estrogens, they can help alleviate some hormonal symptoms, such as hot flashes. Soy protein has real benefits for your heart; eating 25 mg daily can help lower LDL-cholesterol by 5 to 10 percent. You find soy protein in soy milk (7 grams in 1 cup), veggie burger mix (11 grams per cup), tofu (10 grams in 4 ounces), and roasted soy nuts (17 grams in 1 cup), among other foods. (For more information on phytoestrogens, see Chapter 14.)

- Omega-3 fatty acids are found in fish, nuts, flaxseed, tofu, and soybean and canola oils. These essential fatty acids help nourish the hair, nails, and skin, but that isn't their only role in preserving health during menopause. New studies have shown that omega-3 fatty acids offer a number of benefits for cardiovascular health. The American Heart Association (AHA) reports that increasing the consumption of omega-3 fatty acids can benefit people who have preexisting cardiovascular disease as well as those with healthy hearts and circulatory systems—especially when those fatty acids are consumed as part of a balanced diet. The AHA recommends two three-ounce servings of salmon, tuna, mackerel, herring, or other fatty fish every week.

Good Sources of Calcium

What foods give you the greatest calcium boost? Here are just some examples (remember to check food product labels):

Food	Milligrams of Calcium
Nonfat, plain yogurt, 1 cup	452
Swiss cheese, 1 oz.	408
Skim milk, 1 cup	302
Whole milk, 1 cup	291
Sardines, canned with bones, 3 oz.	321
Almonds, $1/3$ cup	114
Kale, cooked, 1 cup	179
Spinach, fresh or cooked, 1 cup	122
Macaroni and cheese, 1 cup	362
Tofu, 1 cup	260
Vanilla ice cream, 1 cup	170

More on Using Calcium and Vitamin Supplements

Some estimates indicate that most menopausal women eat only about half as much calcium as they require each day. And many women have trouble digesting dairy products, so upping their intake of milk, yogurt, and cheese may not be an option for getting the increased calcium their bones demand.

Calcium supplements are available in a number of forms today. Keep these facts in mind when choosing and using calcium supplements:

- The elemental calcium content is what matters most. Check the label carefully to make sure the supplement carries the appropriate amount of elemental calcium.
- Choose calcium supplements from reputable makers; check the label to see if the calcium is purified and look for the USP (United States Pharmacopeia) symbol to help guarantee reliability.
- Calcium works best when you take it in 500-milligram doses, divided over the course of the day.

Most all-purpose vitamins contain a daily dose of vitamin D, as do some calcium supplements. Minerals such as phosphorous and magnesium are important for bone health, too. Again, adequate doses of these are available in most multivitamins.

The Facts about Midlife Weight Gain

As your metabolism slows, you burn fewer calories; as your percentage of muscle tissue decreases and fat tissue increases, your body uses up fewer calories. These facts together mean that, all other things remaining equal, if you continue to consume the same number of calories through perimenopause and menopause that you consumed when you were premenopausal, you can expect to gain weight.

In one study conducted by the University of Pittsburgh, women gained an average of 2 kilograms (about 4.4 pounds) over three years of their menopausal transition. By eight years after menopause, the women gained an average of 5.5 kilograms (a little over 12 pounds). Though all women won't gain this much weight during menopause, many will—and some will gain even more. Without question, exercise is a must for controlling midlife weight gain. (See Chapter 15.) But

How Many Calories Do You Need?

To calculate how many calories you need to maintain your weight, follow these steps:

1. Start with this number: 387.
2. Multiply age by 7.31.
3. Subtract line 2 from line 1.
4. Multiply weight (lb.) by 4.91.
5. Multiply height (in.) by 16.78.
6. Add lines 4 and 5.
7. Enter daily physical activity level:
   Sedentary: 1
   Less than 30 minutes/day: 1.14
   30–60 minutes/day: 1.27
   More than 60 minutes/day: 1.45
8. Multiply line 6 and 7.
9. Add lines 3 and 8.

That number is your caloric maintenance level. (Source: *The Female Patient.*)

eating a healthy, well-balanced diet is your other weapon to fight off this potentially deadly problem.

Women's bodies change during their transition, and the addition of one or two pounds is an expected part of that change. But overweight and obesity—as determined by a Body Mass Index (BMI) of 25 or higher—are conditions associated with all sorts of health risks for men and women alike, including high cholesterol and high blood pressure. The heavier you are, the harder you must work to move, and the less you feel like exercising. Being overweight can make you feel lethargic, depressed, and powerless—feelings no woman needs during her transition through menopause.

The redistribution of body fat to your abdomen and midsection has dangerous implications. A large amount of abdominal fat is considered a high-risk factor for the development of diabetes and coronary heart disease.

Fad Diets Aren't the Answer

Adopting and maintaining a healthy diet does not mean starving yourself or combining certain foods to magically block fat from being absorbed into your system. Long-term weight loss requires you to change your eating habits for good. A healthy diet for long-term weight loss involves common sense: lowering your fat intake, lowering your simple sugar intake, and decreasing your portion size. In general, you must eliminate 3,500 calories from your diet in order to lose a single pound of body fat. By lowering your calorie intake and increasing the number of calories you burn through regular exercise, you will maintain a healthy weight.

Good Eating Habits Aid Weight Control

Good eating habits are crucial to managing weight gain during

Body Mass Index Table

BMI	19	20	21	22	23	24	25	26	27	28	29	30	31	32	33	34	35	36	37	38	39	40	41	42	43	44	45	46	47	48	49	50	51	52	53	54
Height (inches)												Body weight (pounds)																								
58	91	96	100	105	110	115	119	124	129	134	138	143	148	153	158	162	167	172	177	181	186	191	196	201	205	210	215	220	224	229	234	239	244	248	253	258
59	94	99	104	109	114	119	124	128	133	138	143	148	153	158	163	168	173	178	183	188	193	198	203	208	212	217	222	227	232	237	242	247	252	257	262	267
60	97	102	107	112	118	123	128	133	138	143	148	153	158	163	168	174	179	184	189	194	199	204	209	215	220	225	230	235	240	245	250	255	261	266	271	276
61	100	106	111	116	122	127	132	137	143	148	153	158	164	169	174	180	185	190	195	201	206	211	217	222	227	232	238	243	248	254	259	264	269	275	280	285
62	104	109	115	120	126	131	136	142	147	153	158	164	169	175	180	186	191	196	202	207	213	218	224	229	235	240	246	251	256	262	267	273	278	284	289	295
63	107	113	118	124	130	135	141	146	152	158	163	169	175	180	186	191	197	203	208	214	220	225	231	237	242	248	254	259	265	270	278	282	287	293	299	304
64	110	116	122	128	134	140	145	151	157	163	169	174	180	186	192	197	204	209	215	221	227	232	238	244	250	256	262	267	273	279	285	291	296	302	308	314
65	114	120	126	132	138	144	150	156	162	168	174	180	186	192	198	204	210	216	222	228	234	240	246	252	258	264	270	276	282	288	294	300	306	312	318	324
66	118	124	130	136	142	148	155	161	167	173	179	186	192	198	204	210	216	223	229	235	241	247	253	260	266	272	278	284	291	297	303	309	315	322	328	334
67	121	127	134	140	146	153	159	166	172	178	185	191	198	204	211	217	223	230	236	242	249	255	261	268	274	280	287	293	299	306	312	319	325	331	338	344
68	125	131	138	144	151	158	164	171	177	184	190	197	203	210	216	223	230	236	243	249	256	262	269	276	282	289	295	302	308	315	322	328	335	341	348	354
69	128	135	142	149	155	162	169	176	182	189	196	203	209	216	223	230	236	243	250	257	263	270	277	284	291	297	304	311	318	324	331	338	345	351	358	365
70	132	139	146	153	160	167	174	181	188	195	202	209	216	222	229	236	243	250	257	264	271	278	285	292	299	306	313	320	327	334	341	348	355	362	369	376
71	136	143	150	157	165	172	179	186	193	200	208	215	222	229	236	243	250	257	265	272	279	286	293	301	308	315	322	329	338	343	351	358	365	372	379	386
72	140	147	154	162	169	177	184	191	199	206	213	221	228	235	242	250	258	265	272	279	287	294	302	309	316	324	331	338	346	353	361	368	375	383	390	397
73	144	151	159	166	174	182	189	197	204	212	219	227	235	242	250	257	265	272	280	288	295	302	310	318	325	333	340	348	355	363	371	378	386	393	401	408
74	148	155	163	171	179	186	194	202	210	218	225	233	241	249	256	264	272	280	287	295	303	311	319	326	334	342	350	358	365	373	381	389	396	404	412	420
75	152	160	168	176	184	192	200	208	216	224	232	240	248	256	264	272	279	287	295	303	311	319	327	335	343	351	359	367	375	383	391	399	407	415	423	431
76	156	164	172	180	189	197	205	213	221	230	238	246	254	263	271	279	287	295	304	312	320	328	336	344	353	361	369	377	385	394	402	410	418	426	435	443

Normal   Overweight   Obese   Extreme Obesity

menopause. If you want to avoid excess weight gain, the following suggestions may help you:

- Avoid fast food. No matter how easy it is, fast food is packed with all of the things you don't need to eat, such as saturated fats, sugar, cholesterol, and salt. Plan menus, shop for fresh produce, and pack your lunch (with daytime snacks). If you must buy food on the run, order a salad with low-fat dressing on the side and a bottle of water instead of a soda.

- Enjoy your meals. Sit down at a table whenever possible. Shoveling food down while you stare at the television or drive to work is a sure ticket to overeating. Take your time, eat with purpose, chew slowly and thoroughly, and give your stomach time to send signals back to the brain—you'll be more likely to know when you're full.

- Do wait until you are hungry, but don't wait until you're crazed with starvation to eat. Eat small meals spaced out through the day. Eat a light breakfast, have a piece of fruit or a cup of low-fat yogurt midmorning, eat a healthy lunch, have a midafternoon snack, then enjoy a light dinner. If you aren't hungry, don't force yourself to eat just because it's the "right" time of day.

- Avoid eating late at night or right before going to bed. Many people in the United States eat very little during the day, then pack it away from the time they reach home until they go to bed at night—a very bad habit. You're active and at work during the day, so that's when you need your fuel. By the time you go to bed, your body should be ready to rest, and it's hard to do that with a full stomach.

- It may be difficult to reform yourself overnight. Rather than get discouraged, start small—buy thin-sliced whole-wheat bread instead of white, try a new squash recipe, declare a weekly salad night, or skip the cookies and have a handful of grapes. Don't punish yourself about your eating habits—just work to make them better.

- Keep a food journal for two weeks, where you write down everything you eat—most importantly, the quantities! It's essential that you know how much you're eating and how many calories you're consuming. Everything you eat counts—even if you think it's "just a spoonful." Even a crisp green salad accrues hefty calories when you ladle on the dressing; get out the tablespoon, measure how much you use, check the label for calorie count. Weigh it, measure it, write it down.

- Pay attention to portion sizes. A protein serving should weigh about three ounces and be about the same size as a pack of cards. A serving of pasta is around 1/2 cup, not the platterful they bring you in most restaurants. One slice of bread or 1 cup of flaked cereal is one serving. A serving of fruit is 1 medium-sized fruit or 1/2 cup of fruit juice; vegetable serving sizes are 1/2 cup (of starchy veggies like corn or beans) to 1 cup of raw salad, carrots, or celery.

Find Healthy Solutions

When you find yourself turning to food for the wrong reasons—to alleviate loneliness, boredom, fatigue, and so on—stop and think of something that will really help. Call a friend, take a walk around the block, read a book, go to a movie, work in the garden, or write in a journal. Food won't solve any problem other than physical (not emotional or spiritual) hunger.

Sane, Simple Guidelines for Healthy Eating

Putting together a healthy diet doesn't require a Ph.D. in nutrition, a live-in cook, or a personal shopper. It just requires education and a commitment to spend a little more time buying and preparing the right foods. Here's what your food choices should represent every single day:

- Six or more servings of whole grains
- Five or six servings of a variety of fresh fruit and vegetables
- Two or three servings of protein foods such as fish, lean animal foods, beans, nuts, and seeds

With those general guidelines in mind, incorporate these dos and don'ts:

- Limit your intake of fats; total fat intake should be under 30 percent of all calories. Avoid transfats and saturated fats. Fats in nuts, fatty fish, olive oil, flaxseed oil, and canola oil are healthier than are those in animal fats, shortening, and hydrogenated vegetable oils, but they still have calories and should be limited.
- Eat a wide variety of fruit and vegetables with deep, rich colors. Green leafy vegetables, oranges, tomatoes, squash, and blueberries are some of the low-fat, high-antioxidant foods you should include in your diet. Starchy vegetables like potatoes give you less benefits.
- Limit your intake of salt. High sodium levels contribute to high blood pressure, and too much salt actually inhibits the natural flavors of the food you eat. If your usual routine includes salting your food before you taste it, work on breaking it. Also consider a salt substitute, particularly if you are on a sodium-restricted diet.
- Add "meno-healthy" foods into your diet. Remember the benefits of fatty fishes—salmon, tuna, and so on—and eat some twice a week. Add soy to your diet, whether through soy milk, tofu, or roasted soy nuts. These foods are high in nutrients and low in fat.

- Be sensible about caffeine and alcohol consumption. Caffeine has been shown to leach calcium from the body, and it can aggravate conditions such as elevated blood pressure, anxiety, and tension. Consider switching from coffee to green tea—many green teas have only small quantities of caffeine and are rich in antioxidants. Don't drink more than one or two alcoholic beverages a day. Excess alcohol leads to health problems, and alcohol is loaded with calories. Though most health experts agree that wine has antioxidant qualities and can be good for you, keep your consumption low. You'll gain less weight and feel better.

The Raw Facts

If you aren't accustomed to eating raw fruit and vegetables, add them gradually to your diet. If you suddenly load your system with an unusually high level of raw fruit and vegetables, you can have stomach pains, gas, and other gastrointestinal complaints.

Your Own Revolution

As you approach midlife, you have an excellent opportunity to re-evaluate your food choices and adopt a diet that will help ensure a long, healthy, active life. Food is a great joy and an important part of many of our favorite family rituals—you should enjoy eating. Maintaining a healthy diet doesn't require that you demonize every donut or treat each stack of pancakes as if it were a ticking time bomb. It simply means making thoughtful choices about the foods you eat and using food as a means to accomplish your health goals.

You'll never have a reason to regret improving your nutrition. Nothing will ever replace the marvelous health benefits of a well-balanced diet and regular exercise.

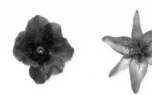

chapter fourteen | **Herbs, Botanicals, and Other Alternative Therapies**

Every woman has a different response to the natural process of meno-pause and the ways it affects her body, her emotions, and often her entire life. Many women choose not to use traditional HRT, and others aren't suitable candidates for HRT as a result of a personal or family medical history. If you are among these women—or are simply interested in learning more about nontraditional or nonprescription treatment options—this chapter provides some good information about HRT alternatives.

Reasons for Seeking Alternatives

Medical complications aren't the only factor that might send a woman in search of an alternative to HRT. Some of the reasons women cite for choosing not to use traditional hormone replacement therapies follow:

- **Troublesome side effects of HRT:** Many women who begin HRT later discontinue its use due to progestin-related side effects, includ-ing vaginal bleeding, breast tenderness, bloating, depression, and irritability. New progestins are now available that differ dramatically from those previously available, so don't forget to discuss new pharmaceutical treatment options with your doctor.

- **Fear of an increased risk of cancer:** Many women fear that estrogen or other hormones included in traditional HRT regimens will increase their risk of cancer, even when they have no personal or family medical history of the disease.

- **Aversion to the "medicalization" of a natural process:** A 1997 survey conducted by the North American Menopause Society found that nearly half of American women surveyed considered menopause a natural process that doesn't require medical management.

Most studies indicate that HRT is safe and effective for most menopausal women. Many women who experience side effects while on HRT find that after a period of a few months, those symptoms lessen or disappear entirely. No responsible medical authority would encourage a woman with a medical history that puts her at an increased risk for developing (or redeveloping) cancer or other diseases and illness to take HRT.

Take Other Precautions if You Don't Use HRT

If you choose not to take HRT for either medical or personal reasons, you need to adopt other means of protecting your bones, brain, heart, and skin as you get older. As you consider alternatives to HRT, it's important that you remember the full range of symptoms and conditions you may need to combat.

The "medicalization" question is one each woman must resolve for herself. Only you can decide whether the potential benefits of HRT outweigh your resistance to replacing your body's naturally diminishing hormones. Really assess your position on this issue; every time you take an aspirin to relieve a headache or use an antibiotic ointment to protect a cut or scratch, you're altering very natural processes. And if you begin a regimen of any herb, pharmaceutical, or supplement to offset the symptoms and physical changes of menopause, you are attempting to manage the process.

HRT might not be the only option or solution for everyone; it's necessary for each individual to look for the approach that works best for her. However, you need to approach any alternative treatment option with open eyes and healthy skepticism.

Be Aware of Effects and Interactions

Plant substances aren't inherently safer or more benign than laboratory-produced chemicals. Plant extracts can be very powerful and can interact with prescription or nonprescription drugs to cause dangerous side effects. Don't take any substance without fully understanding its effects, and ask your health-care provider if it's safe for you. Also don't take more than the recommended dose; tell your health-care professional exactly how much you are taking.

Choosing Natural Alternatives Wisely

You can't walk down the aisle of any grocery, pharmacy, or health food store these days without finding an ever-growing selection of herbal compounds and other so-called botanical or homeopathic treatments that offer a natural approach to better health. An increasing number of botanical supplements are advertised for the management of menopausal symptoms. Some of these alternatives are effective—some aren't. Some can be downright dangerous when taken without the knowledge or advice of a trained nutritionist or health-care professional. Because the sale of herbal compounds and nutraceuticals—

foods that also deliver some sort of medication or compound designed to offer a specific medical benefit—has become such big business, it has drawn the attention of the popular media as well as the medical community.

Information on Herbs

Phytoestrogens, or soy isoflavones, are not true hormones. They are 100 percent natural products made from plants that seem to have the ability to balance the decline in natural hormonal activity that occurs during menopause. Women interested in further information on these and other herbs can visit the American Botanical Council's Web site at *www.herbalgram.org.*

Frequent articles in magazines, newspapers, and on Internet pages discuss the latest vitamin or herbal alternatives, and the scientific community continues to test and release results on the efficacy of these compounds for the treatment of specific physical or emotional disorders. Because botanical extracts, herbal supplements, and nutraceutical compounds aren't inspected or approved by the Food and Drug Administration, however, they haven't passed the rigorous testing process of approved pharmaceuticals, and they haven't undergone a scientifically controlled process of long-term, in-depth study.

Be aware that you can't just stroll down the aisle of your local health food store and choose a safe, effective, natural cure for any of your hormonal symptoms based on the claims of the label (or on other women's experiences you read about in popular consumer magazines or Internet chat rooms). You need to be responsible for making the wisest, most informed choice when buying these products, because a great deal remains to be learned about their safety, effectiveness, and long-term value.

Watch for New Studies

Many of the nonhormonal treatments for hot flashes and other menopause symptoms are controversial, and their effectiveness, safety, and possible side effects and interactions with other medications remain the subject of many ongoing studies.

Herbs, Plant Estrogens, and Supplements

Women have been using herbs to combat the symptoms of menopause for centuries—in fact, only in the past century have any other options been available. As pharmaceutical science has evolved over the past hundred years, so has our understanding of the benefits of supplementing a healthy diet with vitamin and mineral compounds. Today, nearly every woman takes some form of vitamin, herb, or nutritional supplement at some time—if not throughout her life. Most healthcare experts recommend that women supplement a healthy diet with certain vitamins and minerals as they approach menopause.

Use Herbs Cautiously

Certain man-made and herbal dietary supplements should be used with caution, if at all, by women who are postmenopausal. For example, ginseng has a mild estrogenic effect that can cause vaginal bleeding in postmenopausal women—a situation that can easily be mistaken as a symptom of uterine cancer. To avoid potential problems, make sure your doctor okays all dietary supplements.

Many women turn to botanical compounds, plant and herb extracts, and nutritional supplements to alleviate the symptoms of perimenopause and to offset the physical changes the body can experience as a result of estrogen depletion and the natural aging process.

Things to Consider Before Choosing a Supplement

The need for information for women seeking a natural alternative to HRT for the relief of menopausal symptoms is especially critical; the alternatives must offer relief from a range of overt symptoms while, at the same time, supplementing the body's supply of important vitamins and minerals. Consider the following important points when you're assessing the value of choosing herbs and/or nutritional supplements for the treatment of menopausal symptoms:

- **Are you looking for symptom relief or health maintenance?** Many herbal alternatives are effective for relieving a single symptom or for supplementing a specific nutritional need. The wider the range of relief you are seeking, the more pills, capsules, powders, and teas you may need to consume. And you will need your health-care professional to assess the safety of that combination.
- **Have you already adopted the healthy lifestyle changes recommended for women at your stage of life?** No botanical compound, vitamin collection, or nutritional supplement will replace basic necessities such as proper diet, regular exercise, and good stress-management skills to maintain your health through menopause.
- **Have you talked with others who are using the treatment alternative you're considering, and have you discussed it with your health-care provider?** Making a decision to use alternatives requires educating yourself on all of the possible benefits and drawbacks of your choice. Don't think you can tinker with harmless experimentation. Your choice of botanical and nutritional supplements that are powerful enough to treat symptoms and diminish the physical degradation of bone, muscle, and brain tissue that accompanies menopause, without causing risky side effects, is slim. Don't get deluded into thinking that if a health

store supplement is expensive, it's automatically safe and good for you. You may be better off taking prescription medication and paying a small co-pay instead.

The range of botanical substances, nutritional supplements, and nutraceuticals available for perimenopausal and menopausal women is vast. Appendix B contains a number of authoritative references for more information on this topic. The following sections list some of the most popular—and promising—herbs, plant extracts, and nutritional supplements in use today for management of menopausal symptoms.

Phytochemicals

Phytochemicals are chemical compounds found in plants. These compounds are not vitamins or minerals and therefore aren't considered essential for life. As pigments, oils, flavors, and microstructures, phytochemicals appear to work both alone and together, alongside other nutrients in food. They have been associated with the prevention and/or treatment of at least four of the leading causes of death in the United States: cancer, heart disease, diabetes, and high blood pressure. Because there are so many phytochemicals (approximately 4,000), they are separated into different groups.

Certain plants contain phytohormones—natural substances found in some herbs and other plants that may help to regulate the plant's growth. Though plant and human hormones are very different substances, phytohormones (some types are referred to as phytoestrogens) can bind to the human body's estrogen receptors; phytoestrogens may act like an estrogen on the body or like an antiestrogen, depending upon their particular type and dosage.

Found primarily in soy products, phytoestrogens are the plant version of the female hormone estrogen. Researchers are looking at a potential role of phytoestrogens in the fight against cancer, heart disease, and osteoporosis. They're also investigating the use of isoflavones in the treatment of menopausal symptoms such as hot flashes and night sweats.

Vitamin E

In studies where participants took a regulated daily dose of 800 international units of vitamin E, the women did experience some minor relief (on the order of one less hot flash per day), and the vitamin caused no negative side effects. Right now, no study supports the idea that you can achieve significant relief from hot flashes by taking vitamin E, but (again) studies continue in this area. Vitamin E remains a popular supplement, however, for its antioxidant benefits and its ability to decrease breast tenderness, such as women experience with fibrocystic breast disease.

Isoflavones and Lignans

Two of the most popular types of phytoestrogens used in menopausal supplements today are isoflavones (a class of bioflavonoids) and lignans. Isoflavones occur in soybeans, red clover, and (in much lower quantities) green tea, peas, pinto beans, lentils, and other legumes. Lignans occur in flaxseeds (though flaxseed oil contains only small amounts).

What Is a Bioflavonoid?

Bioflavonoids are naturally occurring plant substances found in many brightly colored fruits and vegetables, such as cherries, oranges and other citrus, grapes, leafy vegetables, wine, and some types of red clover. Researchers are studying bioflavonoids for the treatment of a number of conditions, including the control of bleeding, hemorrhoids, and varicose veins.

Natural estrogen can be extracted from some foods, such as soy, and plant hormones from the wild yam have been extracted to create a progesterone-like cream. Some tests have shown that certain plant estrogens offer some relief from hot flashes of perimenopause and menopause, if the symptoms are mild. Taken in normal quantities, they are generally not harmful. They are the subject of a great deal of ongoing research, as the medical community continues to test the safety and efficacy of these substances and to learn how their use compares with the effectiveness of traditional HRT in the treatment of symptoms of women with diminishing levels of hormone production.

Consider Costs

Alternative therapies aren't inexpensive. A recent survey found that the average vitamin/mineral/nutritional menopause symptom treatment costs about $2.00 per tablet—essentially the same as the cost of the usual dose of HRT. If cost is your only problem, investigate some prescription drug discount programs or seek out Internet pharmacies—the cost, especially if you purchase in bulk (usually three-month supplies), is at least one-fourth to one-third less than that at your standard pharmacy.

More on Soy and Isoflavones

Soy is a major source of a number of important vitamins and nutrients, and it is one of the primary sources for isoflavones. Isoflavones are part of the group of phytoestrogen compounds. Although isoflavones are found in a number of plants, only soybeans provide a significant amount of phytoestrogens. While the jury is still out on whether or not soy is as effective as hormone replacement treatment, many experts feel eating a serving or two of soy foods every day can't hurt and may help in most cases. Of course, women who have estrogen-receptor positive tumors are advised to talk to their doctors before adding soy foods or supplements to their diet.

The North American Menopause Society has reported on a number of studies of the use of isoflavones and their role in managing menopausal health. (Some of the articles are listed in the References section of Appendix B.) Though some of the studies have been inconclusive and work continues in this area, many health and nutrition experts believe that soy has major benefits for treating some symptoms of menopause:

- The isoflavones in soy may help reduce LDL cholesterol and triglycerides while increasing HDL cholesterol levels.
- Many women find that soy reduces the occurrences and the severity of hot flashes.
- Some women report that an increased intake of soy isoflavones helps alleviate their symptoms of vaginal dryness, though no long-term study has confirmed this. (Nothing takes the place of estrogen in this area.)

Although, as previously discussed in Chapter 6, some women opt to use the standard hormone replacement therapy combination of estrogen and progesterone, the majority of women choose not to or do so only for a short period of time. Getting phytoestrogens through the diet—isoflavones specifically—may be an acceptable alternative for many of these women.

Keep in mind that the type of soy you consume has a huge impact on the amount of symptom relief you may be able to expect. For example, raw, green soybeans contain the most isoflavones—as much as 150 milligrams per 100 grams of food—whereas soy "hot dogs" or "breakfast sausage" may contain only 3 or 4 milligrams. Read the labels. Most medical experts recommend that if you're using soy to manage menopause symptoms that you consume at least 100 milligrams per day (for 25 to 50 milligrams of isoflavones). Women who are watching their weight may find that this is too many calories to add to their diet and may choose a tablet soy supplement instead.

Although soy products aren't calorie-free, they do tend to be low in fat, high in dietary fiber, and full of a range of important vitamins and minerals. Soymilk, tofu, tempeh, and imitation meat products such as burgers, sausage, and "unchicken" cutlets are just some of the readily available sources of soy. Soy sprouts, soy flour, and roasted soybeans also are rich sources of soy isoflavones.

Food Sources of Isoflavones

Food Sources	Total Isoflavones (mg per 3½-ounce serving)*
Soy flour, defattened	131
Miso	43
Tofu, firm	31
Soy cheese	31
Tofu, regular	24
Soy hot dog	15
Soymilk	10
Soy veggie burger	8
Peanuts	<1

Source: USDA-Iowa State University Database on the Isoflavone Content of Foods, Release 12, 2000.
*mg = milligrams

Because researchers haven't determined how phytoestrogens in soy interact with cancerous cells, these products aren't recommended for women seeking nonhormonal relief from menopause symptoms if they have a personal or family history of cancer. Many studies are under way on the use of soy in the treatment of menopause symptoms, so keep watching for new information, and ask your doctor about the latest developments.

Red clover is the second richest source of isoflavones. Though some herbal teas and compounds include red clover, it's more commonly taken as a plant extract. Very little properly conducted research has been done regarding this herb's effect on menopausal health and counteractions with other medications older women may be taking.

Isoflavones and Cancer

The low breast cancer rate in Japan—where women eat much more soy than women in the United States—has prompted researchers to look at the potential health benefits of soy isoflavones. A number of studies have shown that soy intake is associated with a decreased risk of breast cancer in premenopausal women (not postmenopausal women). Some experts believe that soy may increase the length of the menstrual cycle, which in turn may reduce the risk of breast cancer. However, not all studies support this theory.

Even though isoflavones are weaker than estrogen, many experts feel that isoflavones may help to reduce estrogen-dependent cancers—but this remains to be proven.

Isoflavones and Bone Health

One of the effects of reduced estrogen levels in the body is a decrease in the activity of osteoblasts—the cells that build bone. Two different studies on humans have shown that isoflavone-rich soy protein may increase bone mineral density and reduce bone loss at the spine. And, unlike animal proteins, soy protein does not induce urinary loss of calcium from the body. However, another study showed that isoflavones in postmenopausal women had no effect on bone health. Long-term studies are now underway and may provide a clearer picture of the role of isoflavones in this arena in the future.

When to Supplement with Isoflavones

Currently, there are no formal RDAs for isoflavones, but studies show that 60 to 90 milligrams per day is needed for bone health, 50 to 80 milligrams per day to reduce symptoms of menopause, and 30 to 90 milligrams per day for potential cancer benefits. Approximately three servings of soy foods per day would provide the upper levels of these recommendations, but many experts believe that as little as one serving of a soy food per day may be enough to reap some of the beneficial effects.

Black Cohosh

Black cohosh is perhaps one of the most popular herbal remedies used for the management of menopausal symptoms. Native American women have used its roots for centuries for relief of a number of symptoms associated with menstruation and menopause. The specific means by which it works is still the subject of intense study. Though some products containing extracts of black cohosh claim they can reduce hot flashes by as much as 25 percent, many medical experts feel that data to verify the herb's effectiveness is lacking. More studies are also needed to determine if black cohosh is safe for women with breast cancer and other estrogen-sensitive cancers, particularly if they are on or have recently finished chemotherapy. Side effects of black cohosh include nausea, vomiting, dizziness, headaches, nocturnal seizures, and abnormal bleeding. Black cohosh should not be used during pregnancy, as it may cause miscarriage or premature birth. In menopause or perimenopause, its use is not recommended for more than six months. (According to a handout used at Grand Rounds at Northwestern Memorial Hospital, National Center for Complementary and Alternative Medicine has research underway that indicates potential drug interactions for hypoglycemics, as well as enhanced chemotherapy cytotoxicity—meaning the side effects associated with chemotherapy.)

Black Cohosh and PMS Symptoms

Today, its traditional use for women has been proven by scientific studies. Germany's E Commission reports that black cohosh is effective for treating women's discomforts, from painful menstrual cramps to premenstrual syndrome (PMS) and PMS-related symptoms such as nervousness, irritability, and moodiness.

It's recommended that 40 to 80 milligrams of black cohosh be taken twice daily, depending on the severity of symptoms. You can also make a tea by pouring three cups of boiling water over one tablespoon of the dried root, steeping, (covered) for ten minutes, and then straining.

Gingko Biloba

Many women turn to gingko biloba supplements, extracted from the leaf of the gingko biloba tree, as treatment for the mental fogginess that seems to descend upon them as menopause approaches. Typical dosages of gingko are said to be 40 to 80 milligrams (taken in

The Use of Acupuncture for Treating Menopause

Acupuncture is an ancient Chinese therapy that involves rotating fine needles until they enter the skin at specific points on the body. In a 1995 test reported by the North American Menopause Society in the journal *Menopause*, women treated with both electrically aided and traditional acupuncture showed a significant decrease in hot flashes, lasting up to three months after treatment. The National Institute of Health Consensus Development Panel on Acupuncture issued a statement saying that acupuncture may be helpful in managing conditions such as headache, fibromyalgia, osteoarthritis, and cramps. This alternative treatment option is still being studied for its applications in the management of menopause symptoms.

capsule form) three times daily, although the supplement has not been adequately studied, especially in terms of safety. Most sources suggest taking this dosage for up to twelve weeks in order to feel the effect. Talk to your health-care provider for information about dosage and appropriateness for your symptoms. Remember, like all other herbal supplements, this supplement can interact with other medications: Be careful if you are taking aspirin, NSAIDs, anticoagulants (e.g., coumadin or warfarin), or nifedipene on a daily or regular basis. High blood pressure, fast heart rate, and abnormal bleeding after surgery have been reported.

Use Kava Cautiously

Kava (sometimes called kava kava) has been used for some time to alleviate anxiety and tension, but it must be used with caution.

Originally a plant of the Pacific islands, some natives used kava as an intoxicant. According to the FDA, its use has been linked to yellowing skin and mild stomach upset. Other side effects include restlessness, drowsiness, tremor, headache, dizziness, and liver toxicity.

Keeping Your Eyes on the Prize

As you approach menopause, you may find that you gain a greater appreciation every day of your health and its precious gifts. No one can stop the aging process—and who would want to? But as our bodies change, as the medical profession uncovers new treatment strategies, as science continually works to forge new understandings of our body and its processes, everything we know about menopause evolves. As you evaluate and follow treatment options for maintaining your physical and emotional health throughout this time in your life, remember to keep an open mind, remain curious, and stay informed from the proper sources.

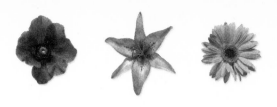

chapter fifteen | **The Importance of Exercise**

By the time they reach the age of perimenopause, most women have developed some strong attitudes about exercise. Either they exercise regularly and can't imagine doing without it, or they've determined that exercise just isn't for them. Exercise combats many of the physical and emotional symptoms of perimenopause and menopause, and—in combination with a healthy, varied, well-balanced diet—it's your best alternative for aging slowly, gracefully, and healthfully.

Why You Need Exercise Now

A woman's body is primed for weight gain in midlife. Although becoming unfit is never a good idea, it can seem particularly damaging at this time. Near the age of menopause, metabolism slows down and muscle tissue diminishes, while fat deposits develop around the center of the body. Hormonal fluctuations can result in a variety of symptoms. Caught in a vicious circle of diminishing fitness, some women find themselves wanting to eat more and exercise less, just when their bodies need the opposite prescription.

Check with Your Doctor First

Never begin any kind of exercise program without first discussing the details with your doctor or health-care provider. Your health-care professional can help assess your capacity for exercise and what type of exercise program might be the most beneficial for your particular needs.

Even those women who maintain the same level of physical activity and food intake through menopause can expect to gain weight and lose muscle tone. This decline in fitness makes even a long-practiced exercise program less effective than it used to be and more difficult to adhere to. In the Healthy Women's Study conducted at the University of Pittsburgh, researchers found that by eight years after menopause, the women in their study gained an average of twelve pounds. The strongest predictor for that weight gain was decreased physical activity.

Does this mean that you're destined for fatness, not fitness, as you approach menopause? Absolutely not! These realities of midlife change simply mean that whatever your current fitness practices may be, they probably need an overhaul when you enter perimenopause. Following are some reasons why you need exercise now.

- Your workday may be less physically demanding than at previous times in your life, and being a "desk potato" doesn't burn any calories.
- Your stress levels may be on the rise because of the demands of your career, family, social, and economic concerns. Stress can cause you to be preoccupied with everything other than exercise, and that will only aggravate weight gain.
- After age fifty, your joint health and physical motor abilities can

begin to deteriorate. The less active you are, the faster (and further) these conditions develop.

- Your body shape and your body image may be changing at menopause. Throwing in the towel on fitness now can set the stage for a continuous decline in health, physical capability, and emotional well-being.

Inactivity Can Lead to Injury

Over 250,000 people suffer from hip fractures every year in the United States. Porous bones, lack of muscle strength, ailing knee joints, and reduced balance and coordination all contribute to these injuries—conditions related to physical inactivity. If you think you're too young to start worrying about these problems, think again. Many women begin suffering from walking impairments as early as age fifty.

Exercise Can Save Your Life

A number of life-threatening diseases become greater health risks for women as they approach the age of menopause. Here are just some of the potentially life-saving benefits of following a regular, sustained program of exercise:

- **Exercise makes your heart healthier:** Regular, aerobic exercise builds the heart and other muscle tissues in the body. The walls of an inactive woman's heart grow thin and are less effective at pumping blood throughout her system, but the walls of a physically active woman's heart grow thicker and stronger. Her heart is healthier and does a better job of pumping nourishing blood throughout her circulatory system.

- **Exercise helps keep cholesterol levels down and arterial flow up:** Even moderate levels of regular exercise can lower the level of LDL cholesterol in a woman's bloodstream. A regular program of aerobic exercise contributes to clean, clear arteries that allow ample supplies of fresh, oxygenated blood to feed the heart and other body tissues.

- **Exercise helps prevent diabetes:** The CDC estimates that diabetes among Americans increased by 49 percent between 1990 and 2000. Obesity and inactivity are recognized as the primary culprits. Numerous studies show that physical activity in combination with a healthy diet can prevent or delay the onset of Type 2 diabetes, even in people who are at high risk for contracting the disease. If you can keep the initial weight gain off, you can avoid that Type 2 predisposition to diabetes.

- **Exercise builds strong bones:** Women who participate in little or no regular physical activity can lose at least 1 percent of their bone mass each year—even before menopause. Participating in regular weight-bearing exercise, including walking, can slow and even reverse this bone loss.

- **Exercise can help prevent some types of cancer:** The American Cancer Society reports that new research has shown that even moderate physical activity can lower breast cancer risk. And, because obesity is considered a risk factor for developing endometrial cancer, exercise helps reduce the risk for that disease. Regular physical activity also reduces risks for developing colon cancer, a growing threat for women age fifty and over.

- **Exercise may help prevent or slow the development of Alzheimer's disease:** A 1998 study conducted by researchers at Case Western Reserve University School of Medicine and University Hospitals of Cleveland found that people who exercise regularly are less likely to develop Alzheimer's disease. Physically active people who do develop the disease are more likely to develop it late in life and experience a slower progression of symptoms.

- **Exercise improves mental well-being in general:** Moderate exercise causes the brain to release more endorphins—naturally occurring substances that resemble opiates. These are the neurotransmitters that make you feel good and happy. The sense of satisfaction that you get from completing an exercise routine will carry over into the rest of your day and may help with the discipline you need to stick to your healthful diet.

Managing Symptoms of Menopause

Beyond the health benefits mentioned above, menopausal women have still more to gain from following a program of regular, sustained exercise. Here's a closer look at some of the menopause symptom-management benefits of exercise:

- **Exercise boosts your metabolism:** As you exercise, your metabolism speeds up, and it remains elevated for a while after you stop exercising. The more energetic and sustained your exercise, the longer the metabolic boost lasts. An elevated metabolism helps your body burn more calories, which can help you lose weight.

- **Exercise may improve cognitive function:** In research conducted at Duke University and reported in the January 2001 issue of *The Journal of Aging and Physical Activity,* regular exercise was shown to improve the cognitive functions of individuals over the age of fifty significantly. Participants who completed thirty minutes of aerobic exercise (walking, jogging, bicycling) three times a week experienced significant improvements in cognitive functions such as memory, planning, organization, and intellectual multitasking. Researchers believe the improvements may be attributed to increased blood and oxygen flow to the brain.

- **Exercise relieves depression:** The original goal of the Duke University study, called SMILE (Standard Medical Intervention and Long-term Exercise), was to determine how regular physical activity compared to antidepressant drug therapy in treating individuals diagnosed with major depressive disorder. After sixteen weeks, researchers found that those participants who practiced the regular exercise program had the same level of symptom relief as did those taking the antidepressant drugs.

- **Exercise helps you sleep:** Many women entering menopause are plagued by insomnia, and countless studies have shown that participating in a regular exercise program can help women go to sleep more quickly and experience fewer sleep interruptions. (Just don't exercise right before going to bed—exercise leaves you feeling pumped up and can make it difficult to fall asleep right away.)

- **Exercise may help prevent hot flashes:** Though no study to date has shown that exercise can stop hot flashes, many studies have shown that hot flashes and other vasomotor symptoms are less common in physically active postmenopausal women than in those who get little or no physical exercise.

- **Exercise improves your endurance and makes you feel like moving:** Regular exercise strengthens muscles, builds endurance, and improves joint mobility and stability, enabling women to remain active and engaged in life.

Your Unique Fitness Goals

Fitness maintenance is your overriding priority now and for the remaining years of your life. If you remain strong, active, and well nourished, you will experience fewer symptoms. You'll have greater resistance to any illness or disease, and you'll progress faster and more successfully through treatments for any condition that does develop.

There is no single universally accepted definition for the term "fitness" because of the vast differences in individuals' genetic makeup. People inherit certain physical characteristics that affect body composition, cardiovascular actions, and other important measures of good health. Heredity also plays a role in how individuals respond to exercise. But your heavy parents or grandparents have not doomed you to being physically out of shape or unresponsive to exercise. The exercise program that's right for your next-door neighbor or even your sister may not be right for you. Your individual hereditary and lifestyle factors determine how your body looks and responds at its peak fitness condition.

Your doctor or health-care professional can help you determine what fitness goals best fit you as an individual. Most health professionals assess fitness based on the following six factors:

- Cardiorespiratory performance or aerobic endurance
- Muscular strength and endurance
- Flexibility
- Body composition—the amount of body fat and its distribution
- Bone density and strength
- Metabolic balance (how the body metabolizes glucose and insulin, blood lipid levels, and other metabolic actions)

Your health-care professional can help you determine healthy goals for your weight, body measurement, endurance, and cardiovascular performance and also monitor your progress and suggest periodic revisions in your exercise program to keep it working for you.

What Kind of Exercise Do You Need?

As unique as your individual fitness markers may be, any complete exercise program includes components aimed at improving three basic types of fitness: aerobic fitness, strength, and flexibility.

Aerobic Fitness

Aerobic fitness involves the functioning of your heart, lungs, and cardiovascular system. Aerobic exercises make your heart work harder, speeding up your heart rate and sending more richly oxygenated blood coursing through your circulatory system to feed all of the tissues of your body. Aerobic exercise has a number of benefits: Among other things, it keeps your weight down, tones your muscles, and makes you feel better about your physical appearance at a time in your life when you really can use a little boost.

Though your health-care provider or fitness consultant will help you determine your specific goals, aerobic exercise is effective when it raises your resting heart rate—your normal heart rate during a period of inactivity—to a target heart rate. This is usually approximately 60 to 75 percent of your maximum heart rate. A treadmill or other fitness test can determine maximum and target heart rates, but you should consult with your health-care provider to help you determine your individual numbers.

Any activity that gets your heart rate up and sustains it for fifteen to thirty minutes is an aerobic exercise, including brisk walking, jogging, swimming, skiing, dancing, bicycling, rowing, hiking, rock climbing, stair climbing, cardio-boxing, power yoga, and a host of other movement-related activities. Remember, most health and fitness experts recommend that you get at least a moderate amount of aerobic activity every day—forty-five minutes to an hour is great. You can break the activity up into smaller chunks of time, if that works better for you. If you can't do aerobic exercises every day, try to do them at least four days a week, even if it doesn't add up to forty-five minutes each and every time.

Warm Up and Cool Down

Whatever type of aerobic exercise you choose, always precede your workout with a five-minute period of stretching and a gradual warm-up toward your full-force aerobic work. At the end of your exercise, spend another five minutes gradually cooling off with, for example, some slow walking or a series of deep-breathing exercises and long, slow stretches.

Variety is key when planning a successful aerobic exercise plan. Changing your routine around challenges your body's muscles to meet new demands and make new improvements. Your commitment to exercise has to last a lifetime, so make it a work in progress by continually evaluating and adapting it to match your growing fitness capabilities, interests, and needs.

Strength Exercises

Health experts today recommend weight training as an important component of the exercise program for all people of all ages. Strength training involves performing a series of repetitive, weight-bearing motions, usually using free weights or some other means of providing resistance against the actions of your muscles. Fixed weight machines, such as the Nautilus line, are available at most gyms and health clubs. Floor work exercises such as push-ups and sit-ups, some yoga postures, and certain Pilates mat work exercises also provide resistance-training benefits for building strength.

Aerobic and Weight-Training Benefits

Aerobic exercises (remember, aerobic means those exercises that boost your heart rate) offer weight-training benefits when your body is upright and your muscles have to support its weight through the exercise movements. Aerobic exercises that include a weight-bearing component such as jogging, walking, step-training, dance aerobics, kick-boxing, and skiing help build strong bones and prevent the development of osteoporosis.

Strength training improves your muscular strength and endurance, of course, but it also helps improve the health and mobility of your joints. It aids balance and coordination, and it builds strong bones—an especially important benefit for women in perimenopause or menopause.

You have a number of options for incorporating strength training activities into your exercise program. Using gym equipment is a great way to ease into resistance training. These machines have adjustable weight levels, and most help you position your body properly to perform the exercises safely and get the maximum benefit from your weight lifting action. A fitness instructor can help you construct an exercise program that includes the use of these machines.

You don't need to join a gym or buy expensive equipment to get a good strength-training workout, however. You can buy a set of inexpensive free weights to do arm curls and lifts at home. (You can even lift cans of soup.) Strap on arm and ankle weights while you clean the house or take your daily walk. Put on your favorite music when it's time to clean the kitchen, and use the rhythm to boost your speed: It will be more fun, the time will go by faster, and, with any luck, the kitchen may come out cleaner. Create a floor-work exercise routine that incorporates traditional exercises such as sit-ups, push-ups, leg lifts, and "air bicycling." Or buy a home-workout video that demonstrates yoga postures, t'ai chi exercises, Pilates movements, or other types of programs that include weight-bearing or resistance-training benefits.

In general, you perform weight-training exercises in sets of repetitions. Most people begin weight lifting, for example, with a weight they can lift six or eight times. (Each lift is a repetition.) You may begin by performing two or three sets of six or eight repetitions, then gradually increase the number of repetitions and the amount of the weight over time. People who want to lose weight but gain muscle tone should do more repetitions using less heavy weights; people who want to increase strength dramatically and bulk up should exercise with heavier weights but do fewer repetitions.

Most medical and fitness experts agree that strength training should make up a smaller portion of your total weekly fitness plan than your aerobic training. Your health professional will help you determine how much (and what kind) of weight-training work is right for you. You may want to include at least one hour of total weight-training time in your weekly schedule. (You can divide that time up into smaller segments.)

Flexibility Training

The length, strength, and elasticity of your muscles and the range of motion of your joints determine your flexibility. Your range of motion may be different from anyone else's—your joints are unique in their intricate makeup and conformation. But your movement patterns and lifestyle habits can determine whether you can achieve the full range of motion your joints are physically capable of or whether you become stiff and inflexible.

Joints require movement and use in order to remain flexible and functional. Movement helps increase the elasticity of muscles and tendons, and it helps stimulate the circulation of blood through the tissues of the joint to keep them well nourished and healthy. Long periods of inactivity allow muscles and tendons to grow stiff; when that happens, your range of motion shrinks, and movements can become awkward and painful.

Resistance Builds Endurance

Strength training works to improve both muscle strength and endurance. The amount of resistance (or the weight you lift or push against) provides the strength-building function of weight training. You build endurance through continued resistance—increasing the total number of repetitions in each workout.

Flexibility is an important quality for any active life. It also contributes to good balance and coordination; if you slip on a wet floor or stumble over an obstacle in the dark, your flexibility may determine your ability to recover your balance and avoid a fall. If you do fall, you'll suffer less injury and recover more quickly if your body is flexible and strong.

Stretching is an important exercise for increasing flexibility. Many exercise practices and programs, including yoga and Pilates, incorporate stretching into most of their exercise movements. Flexibility training typically focuses on shoulders, hips, knees, and the hamstrings (muscles that extend up the back of your thighs). Stretches are slow, controlled movements that gently lengthen and tone the muscles and flex the joints to give them increased elasticity and strength.

Choosing an Exercise Program

It's important that your exercise program meets your physical and emotional needs. You need to enjoy the time you spend exercising; otherwise, you're likely to lose interest in it after a short period of time. The following are some issues to consider.

- Are you better suited to working out alone or does working in a group motivate you?
- How much assistance will you need to begin your program?
- Can you incorporate both indoor and outdoor exercises into your routine to keep it varied and interesting?
- How much money are you willing to spend on gym fees and equipment?
- Is the location of the nearest affordable gym optimal for you?
- Will the program you've chosen be convenient—or even doable—given your schedule?
- Does your program incorporate exercises that will help you build strength, aerobic endurance, and flexibility?

Be open to suggestions and be creative. Hang around with your kids and play catch. Go for a long walk after dinner with a special friend or by yourself. Lift telephone books while you're on the phone. Put on your favorite dance music and hop around while you fold laundry. It's all about getting off your fanny and getting the blood moving again, any way you can. Every calorie you burn, every muscle you flex, every joint you move is a point in your favor. The more you do, the faster those points add up.

Don't give up. Even if you have to step away from your usual exercise routine for a few weeks due to work or illness, get back into it as soon as time and circumstances permit. And don't let weight gain embarrass you into staying away from the gym. You're taking a positive step toward improving your physical condition, and that's something to be proud of. Changes will be gradual, so don't be disappointed if the miracle transformation doesn't happen overnight. Keep at it, and you'll see the results.

Stick With the Program

Walking has the lowest dropout rate of any exercise program. It's free, you don't need a lot of special equipment, and you can do it throughout your life. Most experts recommend walking more than three miles per hour if you're walking for weight loss. (You burn about 240 calories per hour walking at a moderate pace.) But don't forget to mix it up and add other activities to build a complete exercise program.

chapter sixteen | **Breathing and Meditation Techniques**

Meditation is the stilling of all your conscious faculties in order to be present in the moment. It's a powerful tool for keeping your body calm, focused, and strong. Its stress-relieving benefits can help ward off hot flashes and other stress-related symptoms of menopause. Meditation can help to maintain calmness in the midst of things that incite anger; lead you to a deeper understanding of your true self; help you to find serenity and aid depression; enable you to identify your fears and quell them; bring you to accept the reality of a difficult situation; uncover your inner strength; and boost your abilities to deal with stress.

In the past few decades, many professionals have acknowledged the benefits of meditation. In the 1970s, studies on the effects of transcendental meditation, conducted at the Los Angeles Center for the Health Sciences, showed that heart rate, blood pressure, and some endocrine secretions are altered to healthful levels in the meditative state. This effect on so-called involuntary physiological functions is good reason to include meditation in the repertoire of preventive medicine.

Building Your Meditation Practice

In the beginning, you may want to start with exercises that last five to ten minutes and build up a practice from there. Don't pressure yourself or set unrealistic goals. Just stay with your program and you'll progress well.

Learning to meditate doesn't mean you have to adopt a whole new way of being. You can incorporate the benefits of meditation into your present life. Natural postures, movements, and breathing are all that you need to start a meditation practice. You just might have to learn healthier breathing techniques and new sitting positions.

The Similarities Between Prayer and Meditation

Meditation is an innate part of every spiritual tradition, although it may not be named as such. Prayer, contemplation, silence, and ceremony are all meditative acts. They can be found in every religion, ancient and modern, and they are vital to strengthening faith and belief. Both prayer and meditation are essentially the same in spirit and practice. For starters, both share a recognition of the connections among heart, mind, and spirit; a realization that divine energy and grace exists in and around the world of life, and it's accessible to us; a cultivation of qualities of good character; and a discovery of higher power through practice.

Breathing Properly Takes Practice

When you begin to meditate, proper breathing might seem difficult at first. Don't stress yourself out too much over it. Breathing deeply from the abdomen is important, but don't try so hard to breathe properly that you sidetrack yourself and forget what you're trying to do with your meditation. Take things gradually; your breathing will improve with time and patience.

Prayer is an important form of meditation that many people use all the time. Prayer doesn't always have to occur in church—the same kind of focus can be applied in any quiet place. The sort of inner peace derived from prayer is exactly what meditation seeks to cultivate.

Other Common Forms of Meditation

You've probably never realized it, but you often unknowingly enter a meditative state under other everyday circumstances as well. The natural trend toward focus and self-awareness can often come from performing simple, methodical tasks or everyday hobbies (such as knitting) that free the mind from concentrated thought. In these instances it is the realization—without thought or feeling—that you are participating in the moment that brings you into the state of meditation.

Breathe In, Breathe Out

Look down at your stomach when you breathe. It should be going in and out as you exhale and inhale. If your upper body (meaning your chest wall and shoulders) is moving up and down, you are not breathing correctly. Remember: in and out, not up and down.

Body Basics

It makes little difference whether you are able to conform your body to the traditional "lotus" position, sitting cross-legged on the floor. But a few guidelines are necessary for productive and comfortable meditation.

The first and most essential guideline is to allow your spine to be upright and immobile. This position allows for optimum breathing and less strain on the body overall when maintaining a position over an extended period. Nothing should interfere with circulation. The right posture ensures that the entire body can oxygenate without hindrance.

Keep your hands open, palms up; place them downward on your lap or knees or even rest them on your tummy, either folded or interlaced. You can keep your eyes open or closed as you meditate, according to your own preference.

Sitting Postures

You need a firm foundation for sitting postures, but you also need enough padding to promote circulation and comfort. If you decide to meditate while sitting on the floor, you'll need a mat or a cushion to sit on, and you'll have to do some experimentation with the placement of your limbs. If you aren't able to sit cross-legged, a good chair works, too. Remember your feet should be supported—either by the floor, a footrest, or a cushion.

The lotus is regarded as the standard sitting posture of meditation, but there are variations; choose whichever one works for you.

- **Burmese Lotus:** Legs are folded, one in front of the other, so that the calves and feet of both legs are resting on the floor. This is a good beginning posture.
- **Half Lotus:** While seated, just one leg (whichever is more comfortable) is folded upward to rest on the opposite inner thigh. The other leg is tucked under the first.
- **Quarter Lotus:** This is similar to half lotus, except that instead of resting on the thigh, one leg is resting on the calf of the opposite leg.
- **Full Lotus:** While seated, the legs are folded upward, with the right foot placed on the left hip and the left foot placed on the right hip. The hands rest on the knees.

Tips for Good Meditation

Before you begin meditating, keep the following points in mind:

- Maintain a comfortable posture that will not interfere with your concentration.
- Avoid meditating near mealtimes. If you're hungry, a growling stomach may interrupt your meditation session, and if you've just eaten, the digestive process could also be disruptive.
- If you sit in a chair, make sure it's sturdy but comfortable, with a tall back that keeps your spine straight and your back supported.
- Keep your feet flat on the floor and lean back to rest your neck if necessary.
- Avoid tight clothing or footwear, furniture that pushes against your limbs, and slippery fabric covers that will interfere with comfort and relaxation.
- If you sit on the floor, make sure the surface is completely flat, using a rug or pad on hard surfaces.
- Choose a posture that allows you to place your knees as close to the floor as possible so that your spine will remain upright.
- If your back tires easily, lean against a wall with your legs stretched out.

Beginning to Meditate

Meditation begins by focusing your attention on a single point. As soon as you start your first sessions, you may become aware that thoughts and feelings rush forward for your attention. This is because everything you might have put on the back burner bubbles up.

Instead of trying to push those thoughts and feelings aside, incorporate them into your meditation, viewing them in a detached, disengaged manner. If a distracting thought or feeling comes forward, consider what it's communicating to you for only a moment, assign it to its proper place, and allow the next thought to come forward.

Don't get angry or upset if you're feeling restless, impatient, or unfocused. Learning to concentrate on meditation takes time.

Breathing Warm-Ups

Breathing exercises will set the foundation for your meditation regimen. Although you take air into the body through the nose and mouth, when you breathe in meditation, you should use your abdominal muscles, the way babies breathe. It's important to use breathing consciously and optimally, because it contributes so much to physical and mental relaxation.

Deep Breathing During Hot Flashes

If you feel a hot flash coming on, begin taking deep, slow breaths through your nose. Breathe in to expand your diaphragm and abdomen as far as you can; hold the breath for a few seconds, then slowly release it. Let your belly swell out and your chest expand outward as you breathe so your body is fully "inflating." When you exhale, empty your lungs completely. Take at least three full, deep breaths and try to remain calm to diminish the hot flash.

Standing Breath

Stand with your feet slightly apart to balance your weight. Focus only on your breathing for three minutes. Do not attempt to control or direct your breath; just observe it.

Now take three "good" breaths—not necessarily deep or long, just comfortably filling as you inhale and exhale. As you take in each breath, raise your arms; then lower them as you exhale. While inhaling, think of the air also entering your body from the ground upward to your head. Allow each breath equal time in duration and quality. And try not to make it different from the way you noticed your "normal" breathing, especially in the beginning.

Sitting Breath

Sit in a comfortable chair, making sure that you are as upright as possible and your feet are comfortably on the floor, either flat or crossed. Place your hands on your lap or palms down on your thighs. Focus only on your breathing for three minutes. Again, don't try to control or direct your breath; just observe it.

Next, lower your head to your chest, and inhale while slowly raising your head. As you exhale, lower your head back to your chest. Do this for three long breaths, as slowly as possible, without deviating from your normal breathing pattern.

Basic Meditation Techniques

Although there are many types of meditation, there are still some general approaches that apply. Essentially, there are two ways that meditation can be practiced: "with seed" and "without seed." These are generic terms, and just about every type of meditation will fall into one of these two approaches.

Meditation with Seed

In this type of meditation, an image, word, or sound is employed to focus the mind in order to reach the launching point away from ordinary mental activity. In some religious traditions, certain prayers serve as seed meditations. They can be quite extensive, and the entire meditation practice might be based on recitation or the silent reading of such prayers or revered writings. (Saying the rosary is a similar example of this sort of meditative tradition.) In others, words of power or mantras are repeated at length to attain the launching point. Seed meditation can also direct the meditator's focus to images or sounds.

An Easy, Ten-Minute Relaxation

Sit or lie down in a quiet place with your eyes closed. Consciously relax every muscle in your body, beginning with your feet and continuing up toward your head. Concentrate on a single word or object that has personal meaning for you; if other ideas, worries, or mental chatter enter your mind, dismiss them and return to the thought of your focus word. After ten minutes, open your eyes, remain seated, and take three deep breaths before continuing with your day.

Meditation Without Seed

In meditation without seed, the goal is to empty the mind of all its conscious and unconscious contents. This can be accomplished through silence, separation from familiar surroundings, and elimination of all but the basic necessities of daily existence. Monastic life and retreats are an example of this type of meditation tradition. Naturally, meditation without seed is an advanced form. Beginners should use exercises with seed to strengthen mental focus.

Practicing One-Breath Meditation

When you find yourself at a standstill in the midst of what you're doing at work or at home, and you feel as if you've come to the end of the rope you're climbing, stop and take a break for some momentary meditation to refresh and relax your mind.

Pause all thoughts and remind yourself that your inner peace prevails at this moment. Think of that peace as a place within you. Straighten your spine as you do this, and lift your chin upward. Focus your eyes above your head at the ceiling or wall. Take a conscious breath, slowly and deliberately. Think of your place of peace opening its door as air fills your lungs. On exhaling, appreciate the moment for allowing you to pause and return to the work at hand.

Branches of Meditation

Various branches of meditative techniques have grown out of many of the world's great religious and philosophical traditions, such as Yoga, Buddhism, and Taoism. Traditions like these combine religious themes with philosophical approaches, often in the context of the cultural landscapes in which they are practiced.

Other derived practices—such as transcendental meditation, insight meditation, and mindfulness meditation—get to the essence of the process without the cultural details. Whether dealing with stress, a need for healing, or personal growth, the derived meditation practices are advantageous tools, especially if you're looking for an expeditious approach.

Cooling Visualization

When you feel a hot flash begin to develop, close your eyes and envision being in a cool, breezy location. Think of the warmth as a liquid, and imagine that you can channel it to flow from your body. Envision the heat draining out through your hands and feet; as the heat leaves your body, imagine that a cool layer of snow is falling on your head, shoulders, and arms.

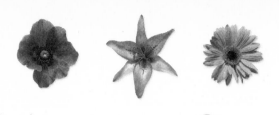

chapter seventeen | **Menopause *Yoga* Practice**

Yoga is an ancient art and science from India, originally designed to strengthen and align the body and quiet and focus the mind for meditation. It's excellent for increasing flexibility, building muscle strength and endurance, and eliminating the negative effects of stress on your body. Practicing yoga stretches for twenty to thirty minutes three times a week can help reduce the negative effects of stress on your body, as it stretches your muscles, improves your balance, and encourages deep, full breathing.

Uniting Body, Mind, and Spirit

The word *yoga* literally means "to yoke or join." Yoga joins and integrates the mind, body, and spirit into one aligned and cohesive unit. In the Western world, most people live in their heads more than in their bodies. It is thought that through the practice of yoga postures and breath work, you can reconnect your body and mind and discover your spirit.

Many people think that you have to be like a Gumby toy—able to touch your toes to your nose—but this isn't true. Everyone can do yoga regardless of age, size, flexibility, or health. Yoga is the great equalizer. Two people can walk into a yoga class, one very flexible with no strength and the other stiff (too strong) with little flexibility. The same poses done by these individuals will tighten up the overly flexible person and loosen the stiff person. There are many types of yoga suitable for anyone and poses can *always* be modified to fit an individual's needs.

The Benefits of Yoga

The yoga postures, known as *asanas*, bend the spine in many different ways, keeping it supple and healthy, and nourishing the entire nervous system. The *asanas* release tension and blocked energy; lengthen and strengthen muscles; and tone, stimulate, and massage the internal organs. As a result, the muscles and organs are bathed in blood, nutrients, and *prana* (life force or vital energy).

Although yoga is fabulous for women of all ages because many of the poses are terrific for the health of the reproductive organs, it's particularly therapeutic for menopausal symptoms. An appropriate yoga practice can alleviate and reduce many of the symptoms menopausal women frequently experience, including mood swings, insomnia, and fatigue. Weight-bearing yoga postures including arm balances, inversions (poses where the head, hands, or forearms are the base, while legs and feet lengthen upward), and standing poses may help to maintain bone density and may possibly even help to prevent osteoporosis.

While it's not possible to cover all of the poses beneficial for menopause in detail within the context of this book, following are some examples. Then, if you're interested in continuing a serious yoga practice, you can take a class. Refer to the end of this chapter for resources.

Basic Poses That Serve as Foundations

Before attempting any of the poses in this section, it is important to learn the proper foundations for a few basic poses. These poses are used often as starting points for many others.

Tadasana

Tadasana, the mountain pose, is the basic standing pose (see Figure 17-1). Like a mountain, you want a broad, stable base from which to extend to the sky. In this pose, you learn how to balance, center, ground, and extend.

Start by placing your feet together, joining the big toes and inner ankles, if possible. Otherwise, stand so the ankles, knees, and hips are lined up, one over the other. When viewed from one side, the ear, shoulder, hip, knee, and ankle should form a straight, vertical line, with your arms by your sides.

Create strong yoga feet by spreading the toes and balls of the feet, pressing into the big and little toe mounds and the center of the heel. Bring the weight a little more into the heels. Lift your arches as you ground the feet. Enhance this action by lengthening your leg muscles all the way up to your hips. Lift the top of the kneecaps up by contracting the quadricep muscle. Firm the muscles of the thigh to the bone.

Now you have created a stable base from which the torso will be able to extend. Place your hands on your hips and extend the sides of the body from your hips to your armpits. This action creates length and space in the spine.

Bring your arms back to your sides without losing the lift of the spine, lengthen up through the crown of your head. Try to balance your head over the pelvis. Make sure the shoulders are relaxed and are

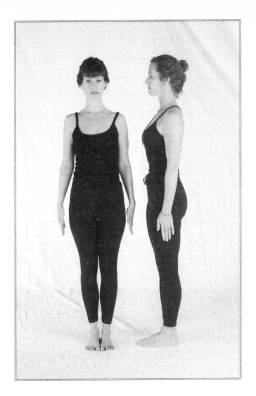

Figure 17-1: Tadasana

not riding up to the ears. Press your shoulder blades into your back. Lift the top of your chest and broaden the collarbones. Breathe fully, and remain aware of how it feels to be in alignment.

Tadasana can be done with your back to the wall for alignment. It can also be performed lying down, with the feet flush against the wall.

Dandasana

Dandasana, the staff pose, is the fundamental seated posture (see Figure 17-2). It teaches the foundation and basic principles crucial to doing seated postures correctly.

Sit evenly on the buttock bones with the legs outstretched and together, in front of you. Place your hands slightly behind the hips and press the fingertips down into the floor as you lightly lift the buttocks off the floor. As you press the fingertips down, stretch the arms up into their sockets. Firm the arm muscles to the bones without tensing the shoulders and neck. This action will stretch and lift the sides of the body and lengthen the spine.

Lightly lower the buttocks to the floor. Press down through the buttock bones and feel the rebounding action going up the torso, lifting and lengthening the spine out of the pelvis. Accentuate this action by extending up through the sides of the body. Move the shoulder blades into the back.

Maintain the pressing down of the fingertips and stretching of the arms to support the torso and elongate the spine. Breathe! Broaden the collarbones and lift the sternum (breastbone), opening the top

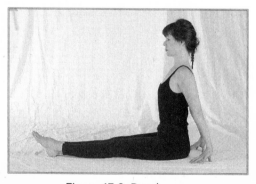

Figure 17-2: Dandasana

chest and keeping the shoulder blades into the back to support the opening of the chest.

Press the back of the legs and the buttock bones firmly into the floor for your foundation. Avoid pressing just the knees down to lengthen the legs, because this creates hyperextension of the knees. The legs must lengthen and extend for the legs to press down onto the floor. Encourage the legs to stretch in two directions. Lengthen the legs into the active yoga feet. Firm the thighs and lift the kneecaps as the thighbones draw into the hip sockets.

Throughout the pose, keep your foot flexed. Have the hands by the hips, fingers facing forward, lightly touching the floor, while supporting the elongation of the spine. Stretch up through the crown of the head.

Gaze straight ahead, reflect, and watch your breath. Stay for several breaths or minutes, depending upon the ease and effort felt in the posture.

You may find it helpful to sit on a folded blanket (or two), to bring the pelvis to an upright, level position to maintain the natural curves of the spine (see Figure 17-3). You can also widen the distance between the legs, or belt the feet while lifting the spine. Or place the hands on blocks.

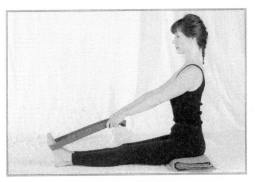

Figure 17-3: Dandasana
while sitting on folded blankets.

Upavistha Konasana

Upavistha Konasana is the seated wide-angle pose. Begin in Dandasana. Separate the legs at a comfortable, wide distance apart. Press the fingertips down by the sides of the body to lift and elongate the torso. Lift the rib cage off the hips. Flex your feet, pressing your heels into the floor. The toes face the ceiling. Actively lengthen the legs in two directions, toward the feet and into the hips (see Figure 17-4). Breathe and be in the pose.

To go farther in the posture, bend forward from the hips and extend the body out and forward. Maintain the elongation of the front, sides, and back of the body. Clasp the big toes or calves with your hands (see Figure 17-5). The buttock bones must remained grounded on the floor. The head may reach the floor or remain.

You can also try sitting on a folded blanket. Place the rounded corner of the folded blanket to face forward. Sit down with the rounded corner under the pubis. This will allow the thighs and groins to release further down to the floor. Wrap a belt around each foot and clasp one with each hand (see Figure 17-6).

Benefits of Upavistha Konasana include: fully stretching the back of the body and the legs, toning the abdominal organs, and improving health of the reproductive organs by increasing circulation. It also balances the menstrual cycle, stimulates the ovaries, and eases menstrual discomfort.

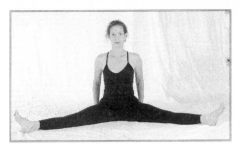

Figure 17-4:
Upavistha Konasana, intermediate

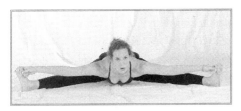

Figure 17-5:
Upavistha Konasana

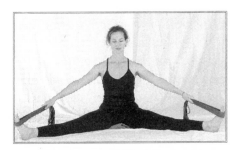

Figure 17-6:
Upavistha Konasana with belts

Adho Mukha Svanasana

Adho Mukha Svanasana is the downward-facing dog pose, one of the most frequently practiced yoga poses. If you've ever seen a dog stretching, you know that this pose looks like an upside down V. Start on the hands and knees (see

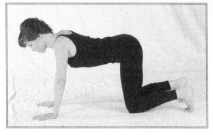

Figure 17-7: Beginning Adho Mukha Svanasana on hands and knees

Figure 17-7). Place the hands under the shoulders and the knees directly under the hips. The inner arms face each other and the elbows are straight and firm. Let the shoulder blades come onto the back. Observe that the upper arm bones connect into the shoulder socket. The pelvis is in a neutral position, horizontal to the floor. Tuck the toes under.

Plant the hands firmly on the floor and spread the fingers evenly apart. Press the palms, knuckles, and fingers into the floor. Especially press down the pointer-finger knuckle and balance the weight on either side of the hand. These are important actions to maintain throughout the pose, because the hands are part of the pose's foundation, and they must stay rooted in order for extension of the spine to occur.

Inhale the breath, lift the hips evenly, and press the hands and feet down (see Figure 17-8). On the exhalation, straighten the legs and let the head drop between the arms. Relax the neck. Press the front of the thighs back to elongate the torso. Press the hands down, extending into the fingertips. Then stretch the arms away from the hand, all the way up to the buttock bones. Let the spine lengthen from the top of the head to the tailbone, into one long line of extension.

Lift the heels up, resisting the shoulders moving forward, and continue stretching all the way up the back of the legs to the buttock bones. Now lengthen the heels down, but keep stretching the back of the legs up (see Figure 17-9). Lift the kneecaps and firm the thighs.

The heels are stretching toward the floor. They might even make it to the floor, but do not force this action if it is not happening. Lift the shins out of the top of the ankles as you press the heels down. The feet are also working, spreading, grounding, with arches lifting to enhance the upward extension of the legs. Fully stretch the legs. Keep the arms as long as possible. Bending the elbows will make it difficult to transfer the weight of the body from the arms to the legs. Remain in the pose for several breaths, extending the spine on the inhalation. Then bend the knees and come down.

You can put the back of the heels against the wall for extra grounding. Or try placing the hands and feet wider apart than shoulder width. This helps ease tight shoulders and hips and is a good way to start practicing downward-facing dog. If the hamstrings are tight, keep the knees slightly bent and focus on lengthening the spine and drawing the tailbone up and back. As time goes on and the hamstrings loosen, fully stretch the legs.

If you have wrist problems, you can put a rolled-up washcloth under the wrists to bring the weight into the knuckles and fingers and take pressure off the wrists.

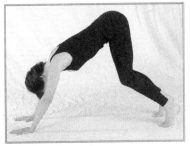

Figure 17-8:
Lengthening the legs

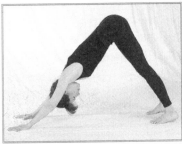

Figure 17-9:
Lifting the hips

Virabhadrasana II

Virabhadrasana II is a warrior pose. Warrior poses create strength of body and mind. Inhale and jump or walk the feet wide apart. Lift and extend the arms out to the sides from the center of the body to the fingertips throughout the pose. Open and lift the chest as you inhale. Keep the chest expanded and lifted throughout the pose (without protruding the front ribs). Turn the left foot in 15 degrees and revolve the right leg out 90 degrees, heel in line with heel. Press the feet firmly down.

Inhale the breath and create extension in the body from the feet up to the fingertips. Exhale fully and bend the right leg to a 90-degree angle, with the knee over the ankle. The entire leg bends to achieve this, not just the knee. The hip, knee, and ankle bend. The right thigh descends down toward the floor. (If you cannot get into a 90-degree angle, don't worry, just do the best you can without force or strain.) As the right leg bends, the left leg remains long. The left foot actively grounds, especially on the outer edge of the foot. The left kneecap lifts up as the quadricep muscle contracts.

There is a dynamic interplay and balance between the action of the legs. As much as the right leg bends, that's how much the left leg straightens through extension and grounding. Become aware of this duality and try to maintain a balance between the two actions.

The arms continue to extend out from the centerline

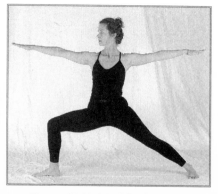

Figure 17-10: Virabhadrasana II

of the body with the shoulder blades pressing into the back, supporting the upper body (see Figure 17-10). The body remains centered between the legs. To achieve this, stretch even more into the left arm and fingertips, so the body remains upright.

The tendency is for the body to lean toward the bent leg. This causes undue strain to the right knee. Imagine that someone is holding onto your left hand and pulling you out of the pose.

Maintain the length and extension of the torso. Lift the ribcage away from the hips, and descend the hips. Feel the space created in the abdomen and the lower back. Gaze toward your right hand and remain for several breaths. To come out of the pose, look forward, press down into your right foot, and lift the kneecap and quadricep up to lengthen the right leg, turn the feet parallel. Repeat on the other side.

You can also practice this pose while sitting on a chair. Bend the right leg out to the side and slide the thigh to the left, so the right thigh is completely supported on the chair. The left leg is now off the chair. Extend the left leg out to the side, grounding and spreading the foot, and lifting the arches. Lift through the sides of the body as you extend the arms out to the sides (see Figure 17-11). Repeat on the other side. If you prefer, you can stand with your back to the wall for support and alignment. Place back outer heel against wall for stability and support.

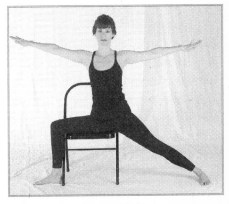

Figure 17-11:
Virabhadrasana II, using a chair

The Basic Relaxation Pose

Savasana is the basic relaxation pose in yoga. In this posture, you learn the art of stillness of the mind and the body. It is typically done at the end of an asana practice in a reclining position.

When the body is systematically relaxed, it allows the mind to let go of the noisy thoughts that cloud perception and prevent total relaxation. During deep relaxation, you are practicing and refining pratyahara, or withdrawal of the senses. This inward focus is essential to turning off external stimulation and enhancing relaxation.

In Savasana, your eyes are closed and your breath is smooth and natural. Deep relaxation occurs while remaining conscious and aware of the entire process. Your mind observes the relaxation process as a witness. You watch noisy thoughts dispassionately as they come in and out of your consciousness, much as you would view a movie screen.

The practice of Savasana also prepares the mind and body for pranayama (breathing techniques).

Performing Savasana

To practice Savasana, lie down with your legs extended and comfortable. Turn your palms up while externally rotating your upper arms. Have your arms rest slightly away from the sides of your body, allowing the armpit and sides of the body to feel open and soft, rather than hard and tense. (As an experiment, bring your arms right next to the body and feel the lack of softness and openness in these areas. Then bring the arms a little away from the body and feel the difference.) Use a folded blanket under the head and neck, so the forehead and chin are level with each other (see Figure 17-12). Balance the sides of the body, arms, and legs, feeling equal weight on the shoulders, buttocks, arms, and legs. Then release the effort. Inhale and exhale deeply, as if sighing, to release the body down to the floor. Remain in

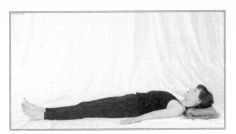

Figure 17-12:
Classic Savasana

this position throughout Savasana, with as little movement or disturbance as possible.

Begin scanning your body systematically, becoming aware of
how you feel. Notice the quality of your breath becoming smooth,
even, and natural. Soften your eyes. Spread and soften your forehead
skin and release your temples. Soften and spread your eyelid skin.
From the bridge of your nose to the center of your eyes, let the skin
spread laterally to the hairline. Feel the heaviness of the front of your
brain, full of noisy thoughts. Soften and release the front of the brain
toward the back of the brain.

Soften your ears deep into the canal and relax the eardrums. Relax
behind your cheekbones as you soften the cheek muscles. Melt the inside
of your cheeks. Soften and spread your chin. Relax the throat muscles
and soften the tongue. Allow your lips to touch and not touch.

Observe the heaviness of your body, arms, and legs as your body
begins to relax and let go. Soften the palms and fingers, the soles of
the feet, and the toes. Relax the diaphragm and soften the front ribs.
Soften your abdomen and release your lower back down to the floor.

Continue to release and soften. Relax your skin down to the
deepest levels. Release the muscles down to their deepest levels. Feel
the heaviness of your bones as they rest completely on the floor.

Observe yourself, very slowly but systematically scanning the body. If your mind starts to drift, gently lead it back. As you continue to lie in Savasana, observe that the earlier heaviness of the body is no longer as noticeable. There may be a floating sensation with the body feeling lighter. Remain in Savasana anywhere from five to twenty minutes.

Then begin to deepen the next exhalation and lengthen the following inhalation, while keeping the brain quiet. Move your fingers and toes and stretch your arms up over your head. Bend your knees and slowly roll onto your right side. Keep your eyes closed, press your hands down, and use your arms to come up to a seated position. Let your head come up last, to maintain a state of deep relaxation. Slowly open your eyes and keep them soft and diffused. See if you can retain the inner focus and calm you have created.

You can also practice Savasana with a bolster or a rolled blanket under your knees or resting your calves on a chair seat. You may want to place an eye bag over the eyes or stay warm by covering yourself with a blanket. Do not do Savasana if you're suffering from depression, mental illness, or phobias, unless the chest is raised and supported.

Savasana can be practiced following an asana practice or anytime you feel stressed out or fatigued.

Learning More about Yoga

If you're interested in learning more about all of the poses in this series and about yoga in general, check out the following Web sites for information and resources for finding classes in your area: *Yoga Journal* (*www.yogajournal.com*); The Yoga Site (*www.yogasite.com*); YogaFinder Online (*www.yogafinder.com*); or Yoga Directory (*www.yogadirectory.com*).

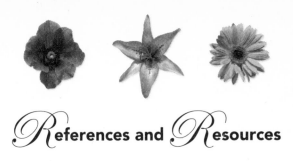

References and Resources

Print and Online Articles, Journals, and Magazines

American College of Obstetricians and Gynecologists. "A Healthy Diet." ACOG Patient Education pamphlet number AP151, ACOG, Washington, D.C.

American Council on Exercise. "Don't Deprive Yourself of the Rewards of Exercise." The American Council on Exercise Fit Facts, online, *www.acefitness.org.*

American Heart Association. "Risk Factors and Coronary Heart Disease." American Heart Association Scientific Position, November 26, 2001.

Association of Reproductive Health Professionals. "Mature Sexuality: Disorders of Desire and Alternative Approaches." ARHP Clinical Proceedings, electronic edition, December 1999, online, *www.arhp.org*

Association of Reproductive Health Professionals. "Perimenopause Update." ARHP Clinical Proceedings, electronic edition, August 2000, online, *www.arhp.org*

Bakos, Susan Crain. "From Lib to Libido: How Women Are Reinventing Sex for Grownups," *Modern Maturity Magazine*, Sept./Oct. 1999.

Brzezinski, Amnon, et al. "Short-Term Effects of Phytoestrogen-Rich Diet on Postmenopausal Women." *Menopause: The Journal of the North American Menopause Society* 4, no. 2 (1997): 89–94.

Carandang, Jennifer, et al. "Recognizing and Managing Depression in Women throughout the Stages of Life." *Cleveland Clinic Journal of Medicine*, 67, no. 5 (2000): 329–338.

Carpenter, Siri. "Does Estrogen Protect Memory?" by Siri Carpenter, *Monitor on Psychology* 32, no. 1 (2001).

"Estrogen Lifts Mood in the Perimenopause," *Women's Health Weekly News*, reprinted in *Health & Sexuality*, Winter 2001.

Fisher, Linda. AARP/Modern Maturity Sexual Survey conducted by NFO Research, Inc. Washington, D.C.: AARP, 1999.

Guthrie, Janet R., and Lorraine Dennerstreing. "Weight Gain, Somatic Symptoms, and the Menopause." *Menopausal Medicine* 9, no. 3 (2001).

"Health for Life," a special issue of *Newsweek* magazine, Fall/Winter 2001.

Harnack, Lisa J., Dr.PH; Rydell, Sarah A., MPH, and Stang, Jamie, PhD. "Prevalence and Use of Herbal Products by Adults in the Minneapolis/St. Paul, Minn. Metropolitan Area." Mayo Clinic Proceedings 2001. July 2001, vol. 26, no. 7.

Holman, Marcia. "Managing the Lesser-Known Effects of Estrogen Loss." MedscapeHealth, online, *www.health.medscape.com*.

Jacobs Institute of Women's Health Expert Panel on Menopause Counseling "Guidelines for Counseling Women on the Management of Menopause." Jacobs Institute of Women's Health, online, *www.jiwh.org*.

Kahn, David A., et al. "Depression during the Transition to Menopause: A Guide for Patients and Families," in *Expert Consensus Guideline Series, A Postgraduate Medicine Special Report*. New York: The McGraw-Hill Companies, Inc., 2001.

Krauss, Ronald M. "Diet and Cardioprotection: Sorting Fact From Fiction." *Menopause Management* 11, no. 1 (2002).

Kurtzweil, Paula. "Lessening the Pressure: Array of Drugs Tames Hypertension." *FDA Consumer Magazine*, July–August 1999.

Mayo Foundation for Medical Education and Research. "Headline Watch: New Evidence of ERT Risks," online, *www.MayoClinic.com*, March 23, 2001.

McNagny, Sally E., et al. "Personal Use of Postmenopausal Hormone Replacement Therapy by Women Physicians in the United States." *Annals of Internal Medicine* 127 (1997): 1093–1096.

"Menopause." On the Alternative Medicine Channel, a member of HealthCommunities.com, online, *www.alternativemedicinechannel.com*.

Menopause Guidebook. Cleveland, OH: North American Menopause Society, 2001.

Murphy, Penelope, ed. *The American College of Obstetricians and Gynecologists Guide to Managing Menopause*. Washington, D.C.: ACOG, 2001.

Newton, K. M., et al. "Women's Beliefs and Decisions About Hormone Replacement Therapy." *Journal of Women's Health* 6 (1997): 459–65.

"Physical Activity and Health: A Report of the Surgeon General." Center for Disease Control online fact sheet, *www.cdc.gov*.

"The Role of Isoflavones in Menopausal Health." Consensus Opinion of the North American Menopause Society. *Menopause: The Journal of the North American Menopause Society* 7, no. 4 (2000): 214–229.

Ryan-Haddad, Ann, and Nasrin Piri. "What Options Exist for Postmenopausal Breast Cancer Survivors with Hot Flashes?" *U.S. Pharmacist* 24, no. 9 (1999).

Scheiber, Michael D., et al. "Dietary Inclusion of Whole Soy Foods Results in Significant Reductions in Clinical Risk Factors for Osteoporosis and Cardiovascular Disease in Normal Postmenopausal Women." *Menopause: The Journal of the North American Menopause Society* 8, no. 5 (2001): 384–392.

Smyth, J., et al. "Effects of Writing about Stressful Experiences on Symptom Reduction in Patients with Asthma or Rheumatoid Arthritis." *Journal of the American Medical Association* 281 (1999): 1304–1309.

"Stealing Time," notes on the film by John Rubin and Ann Tarrant, PBS Online, *www.PBS.org.*

Still, Christopher D. "Health Benefits of Modest Weight Loss." Healthology Press, online, *www.ABCNews.com.*

Takanishi, Gayle C. "Drug Therapies for Hot Flashes in Breast Cancer Survivors." *Women's Health in Primary Care* 3, no. 11 (2000).

"Therapeutic Options During Perimenopause and Beyond." Section G of the Menopause Core Curriculum Study Guide, presented by the North American Menopause Society.

"Too Hot to Handle: Sex and Women over Fifty," in *Vitality: Health and Wellness for Midlife and Beyond*, online, *www.menopausehealth.com.*

Utian, Wolf H., and Pamela P. Boggs. "The North American Menopause Society 1998 Menopause Survey. Part I: Postmenopausal Women's Perceptions about Menopause and Midlife." *Menopause: The Journal of the North American Menopause Society* 6, no. 2 (1999): 122–128.

Weinstein, Sheryl. "New Attitudes Towards Menopause." *FDA Consumer Magazine*, March 1997 (revised February 1998).

"What Is Perimenopause," on Menopause Online, *www.menopause-online.com.*

Wyon, Y., et al. "Effects of Acupuncture on Climacteric Vasomotor Symptoms, Quality of Life, and Urinary Excretion of Neuropeptides among Postmenopausal Women." *Menopause: The Journal of the North American Menopause Society* 2, no. 1 (1950): 3–12.

Other Books on Menopause and Women's Health

DeAngelis, Lissa, and Molly Siple. *Recipes for Change*. New York: Dutton Books, 1996.

Goldstein, Steven R., and Laurie Ashner. *The Estrogen Alternative*. New York: G.P. Putnam and Sons, 1998.

Greer, Germaine. *The Change: Women, Aging, and the Menopause*. New York: Alfred A. Knopf, 1992.

Moquette-Magee, Elaine. *Eat Well for a Healthy Menopause*. New York: John Wiley and Sons, Inc., 1996.

Northrup, Christiane. *The Wisdom of Menopause: Creating Physical and Emotional Health and Healing During the Change*. New York: Bantam Doubleday Dell, 2001.

Sheehy, Gail. *The Silent Passage: Menopause*, rev. ed. Random House, 1998.

Slupik, Ramona. *The American Medical Association's Complete Guide to Women's Health*. Random House, Inc., 1996.

Professional Organizations and Informational Resources

*The American Association of Retired
Persons (AARP)*
601 E Street NW
Washington, D.C. 20049
www.aarp.org

The American Cancer Society
800-ACS-2345
www.cancer.org

*American College of Obstetricians
and Gynecologists (ACOG)*
409 12th Street SW, PO Box 96920
Washington, D.C. 20090-6920
202-638-5577
www.acog.org

American Diabetes Association
1701 North Beauregard Street
Alexandria, VA 22311
800-342-2383
www.diabetes.org

The American Heart Association
7272 Greenville Avenue
Dallas, TX 75231
800-AHA-USA1
www.americanheart.org

The American Lung Association
61 Broadway, 6th Floor
New York, NY 10006
212-315-8700
www.lungusa.org

The American Menopause Foundation
350 Fifth Avenue, Suite 2822
New York, NY 10118
212-714-2398
www.americanmenopause.org

The American Psychiatric Association
1000 Wilson Blvd., Suite 1825
Arlington, VA 22209-3901
888-357-7924
www.psych.org

*The Association of Reproductive
Health Professionals (ARHP)*
2401 Pennsylvania Avenue NW,
Suite 350
Washington, D.C. 20037
202-466-3845
www.arhp.org

Food and Nutrition Information Center
Agricultural Research Service,
USDA
National Agricultural Library,
Room 105
10301 Baltimore Avenue
Beltsville, MD 20705-2351
301-504-5719
www.nal.usda.gov/fnic

National Association for Continence
P.O. Box 1019
Charleston, SC 292402-1019
800-BLADDER
www.nafc.org

The National Cancer Institute
NCI Public Inquiries Office
Suite 3036A
6116 Executive Boulevard,
MSC8322
Bethesda, MD 20892-8322
800-4-CANCER
www.nci.nih.gov

*The National Center for Complementary and Alternative Medicine
(NCCAM)*
NCCAM Clearinghouse
P.O. Box 7923
Gaithersburg, Maryland 20898
Toll Free: 888-644-6226
www.nccam.nih.gov

*National Institute of Diabetes
and Digestive and Kidney Diseases
(NIDDK)*
NIDDK, NIH, Building 31,
Room 9A04
31 Center Drive, MSC 2560
Bethesda, MD 20892-2560
www.niddk.nih.gov

National Menopause Foundation
800-MENO-ASK

National Osteoporosis Foundation
1232 22nd Street NW
Washington, D.C. 20037-1292
202-223-2226
www.nof.org

The National Sleep Foundation
1522 K Street NW, Suite 500
Washington, D.C. 20005
202-347-3471
www.sleepfoundation.org

*The North American Menopause
Society*
P.O. Box 94572
Cleveland, OH 44101
440-442-7550
www.menopause.org